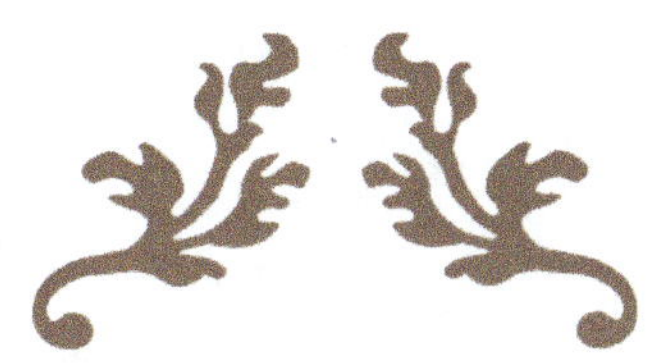

DASH DIET COOKBOOK 2024 EDITION

Delicious Healthy Recipes to Lower Blood Pressure

Dr. Julie S. Clay

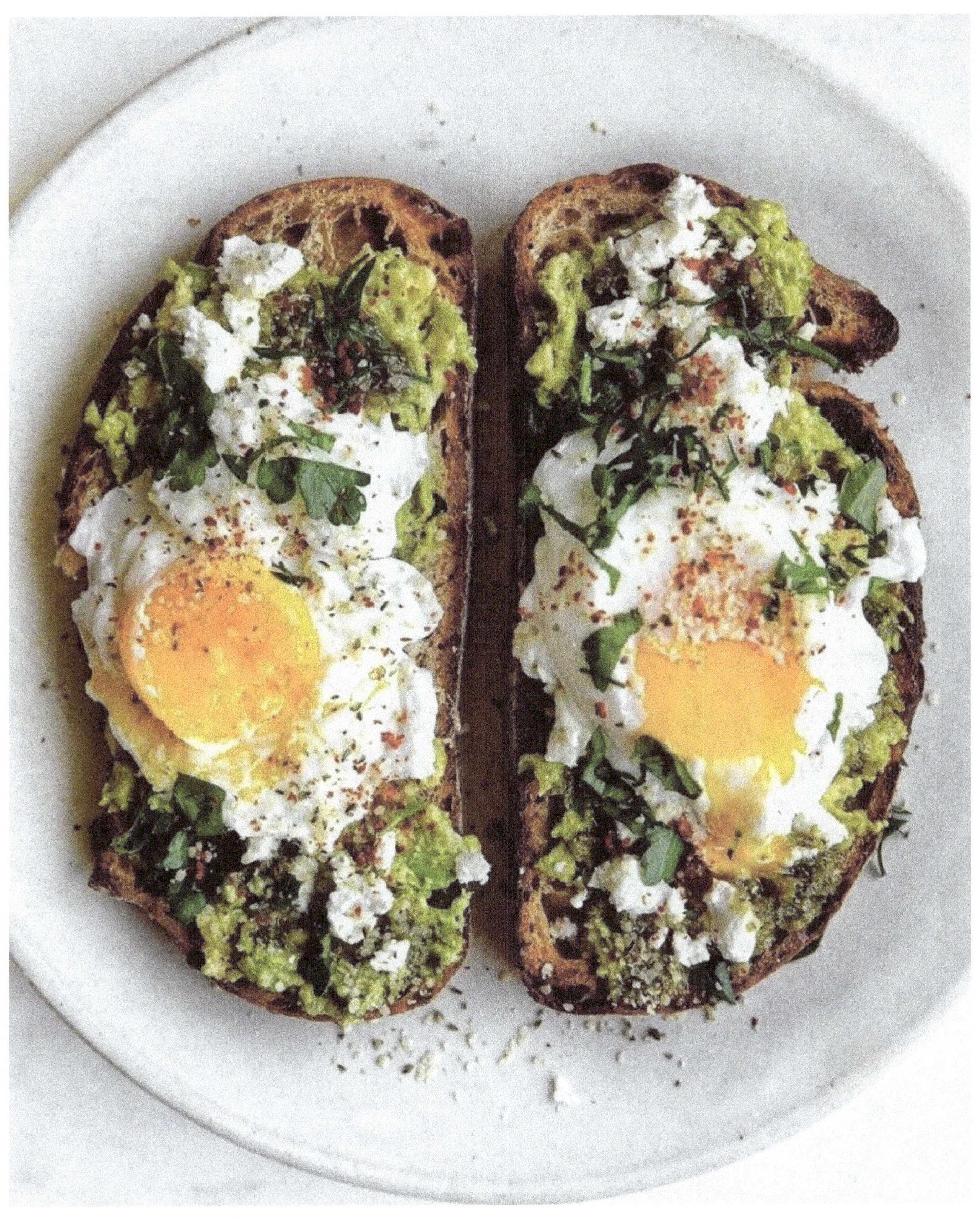

Content

Introduction..4

   The DASH Diet Explained..5

   Key Principles of the DASH Diet...5

   Benefits of the DASH Diet...6

   How to Use This Cookbook...6

Breakfast Recipes...8

Lunch Recipes...22

Dinner Recipes..37

Snacks and sides...51

Dessert Recipes...65

Beverages..79

30-Day Meal Plan..91

Conclusion..94

   Bringing It All Together...95

   Recap of DASH Diet Benefits...95

   Tips for Sustained Success..95

   Final Thoughts and Encouragement...96

Introduction

Dr. Julie S. Clay

The DASH Diet Explained

The DASH (Dietary Approaches to Stop Hypertension) diet is a well-researched eating plan developed to combat high blood pressure (hypertension) and improve heart health. Originally formulated through research funded by the National Institutes of Health (NIH), the DASH diet emphasizes the consumption of whole foods that are rich in essential nutrients, such as potassium, calcium, magnesium, and fiber, while reducing the intake of sodium, saturated fats, and added sugars.

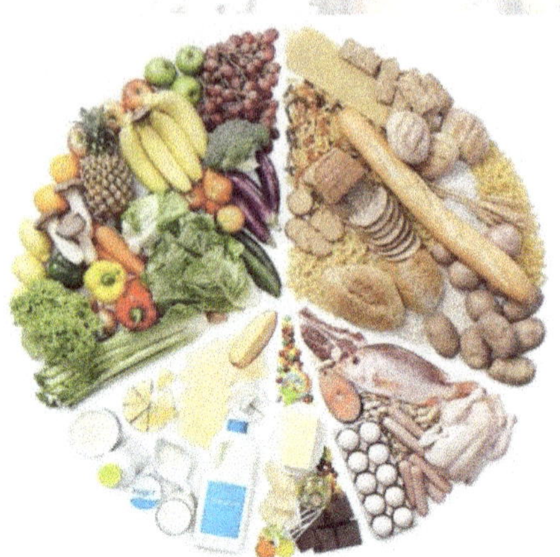

Key Principles of the DASH Diet

High Intake of Fruits and Vegetables: Fruits and vegetables are rich in essential vitamins, minerals, and fiber. They help to reduce blood pressure by providing potassium and magnesium, which counterbalance the effects of sodium.

Whole Grains: Whole grains are a significant source of fiber and nutrients. They help improve digestion, control blood sugar levels, and provide sustained energy.

Low-Fat Dairy Products: These are important for providing calcium and vitamin D without the added fats found in whole milk products.

Lean Proteins: Lean meats, fish, poultry, and plant-based proteins like beans and nuts are encouraged. These sources supply all the necessary amino acids without having too much saturated fat.

Reduced Sodium Intake: The diet aims to keep sodium consumption below 2,300 milligrams per day, ideally reducing it to 1,500 milligrams for those who need to lower their blood pressure significantly.

Limited Saturated Fats and Cholesterol: By focusing on healthy fats from fish, nuts, and vegetable oils, the diet helps to manage cholesterol levels and promote heart health.

Moderate Amounts of Nuts, Seeds, and Legumes: These foods provide healthy fats, protein, and fiber, contributing to satiety and heart health.

Benefits of the DASH Diet

The DASH diet is praised for its numerous health benefits, which extend beyond blood pressure control. The following are a few of the main benefits:

Lower Blood Pressure: Numerous studies have shown that the DASH diet effectively lowers systolic and diastolic blood pressure. This reduction is significant even for individuals with normal blood pressure, promoting overall cardiovascular health.

Weight Management: By focusing on nutrient-dense foods that are naturally lower in calories, the DASH diet helps with weight loss and maintenance. It encourages fullness and lessens the chance of overindulging.

Reduced Risk of Heart Disease: The diet's emphasis on whole foods, healthy fats, and low sodium intake helps to lower LDL (bad) cholesterol levels, reducing the risk of heart disease and stroke.

Improved Insulin Sensitivity: The high fiber content and balanced nutrient profile of the DASH diet help regulate blood sugar levels, making it beneficial for individuals with or at risk of developing type 2 diabetes.

Enhanced Nutritional Intake: By prioritizing fruits, vegetables, whole grains, and lean proteins, the DASH diet ensures a well-rounded intake of essential nutrients, improving overall health and vitality.

Cancer Prevention: Some studies suggest that the high intake of antioxidants from fruits and vegetables on the DASH diet may help reduce the risk of certain cancers.

How to Use This Cookbook

This cookbook is designed to be your comprehensive guide to preparing delicious, nutritious meals that align with the DASH diet principles. Here's how to make the most of it:

Organization and Structure

Section Breakdown: The cookbook is divided into sections by meal type: Breakfast, Lunch, Dinner, Snacks and Sides, Desserts, and Beverages. Each section contains a variety of recipes tailored to different tastes and dietary needs.

Nutritional Information: Each recipe includes detailed nutritional information, allowing you to monitor your intake of calories, sodium, fats, proteins, and other key nutrients.

Recipe Instructions

Step-by-Step Guidance: Recipes are written with clear, concise instructions to guide you through the preparation and cooking process. This ensures that even novice cooks can successfully prepare these meals.

Cooking Tips: Look for tips and tricks throughout the cookbook that provide additional insights, substitutions, and variations to suit your preferences or dietary restrictions.

Meal Planning and Preparation

Weekly Meal Plans: Utilize the sample meal plans provided to organize your weekly meals. This helps streamline grocery shopping and ensures you stay on track with your DASH diet goals.

Batch Cooking and Storage: Some recipes include instructions for batch cooking and storage, making it easier to prepare meals in advance and enjoy home-cooked food even on busy days.

Essential DASH Diet Ingredients

To fully embrace the DASH diet, stocking your kitchen with the right ingredients is crucial. Here's a list of essential items you'll need:

Fruits and Vegetables

Fruits: Apples, bananas, berries, citrus fruits, melons, peaches, pears, and grapes.

Vegetables: Leafy greens (spinach, kale, collards), broccoli, carrots, tomatoes, peppers, cucumbers, and squash.

Whole Grains

Grains: Brown rice, quinoa, bulgur, barley, whole wheat pasta, and whole grain bread.

Cereals: Look for whole grain cereals with minimal added sugars.

Lean Proteins

Meats: Skinless chicken, thinly sliced beef and pork.

Seafood: Salmon, tuna, mackerel, and other fatty fish rich in omega-3 fatty acids.

Plant-Based: Beans, lentils, chickpeas, tofu, and tempeh.

Dairy

Low-Fat Options: Skim milk, low-fat yogurt, and reduced-fat cheese.

Healthy Fats

Oils: Canola, avocado, and olive oils.

Nuts and Seeds: walnuts, chia seeds, flaxseeds, sunflower seeds, and almonds.

Spices and Herbs

Seasonings: Fresh and dried herbs (basil, oregano, rosemary), garlic, ginger, and spices (turmeric, cinnamon, cumin).

Beverages

Healthy Drinks: Water, herbal teas, and occasional servings of 100% fruit juice without added sugars.

By following this cookbook and incorporating these essential ingredients, you can enjoy a diverse range of flavorful meals while reaping the numerous health benefits of the DASH diet. Whether you're a seasoned chef or new to cooking, this guide will help you maintain a nutritious, heart-healthy diet with ease.

Dr. Julie S. Clay

Breakfast Recipes

Breakfast is often considered the most important meal of the day, setting the tone for your energy levels and mood. In the DASH Diet Cookbook, our breakfast recipes are designed to provide a nutritious, satisfying start to your day, packed with the essential nutrients needed to fuel your morning activities and maintain optimal health. These recipes emphasize whole grains, lean proteins, fresh fruits, and vegetables, aligning with the DASH diet principles to help you manage blood pressure, maintain a healthy weight, and support overall well-being. From hearty overnight oats and protein-rich wraps to fresh fruit parfaits and nutrient-dense quinoa bowls, our breakfast selection offers a variety of delicious and easy-to-prepare options to suit all tastes and lifestyles. Dive into these recipes to kickstart your day with wholesome, heart-healthy meals that will keep you energized and ready to tackle whatever comes your way.

Blueberry Almond Overnight Oats

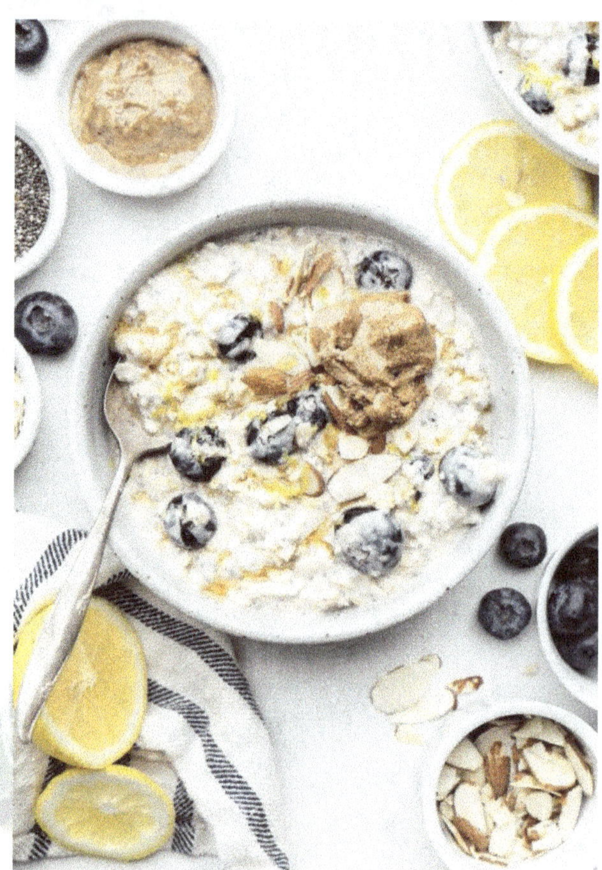

Blueberry Almond Overnight Oats are a perfect breakfast option for those who need a quick, nutritious start to their day. This recipe is packed with fiber, protein, and healthy fats, providing sustained energy and satiety. Overnight oats are incredibly convenient as they require no cooking and can be prepared the night before, making your morning routine smoother and more efficient.

Preparation Time and Serving Units

Preparation Time: 10 minutes

Chill Time: 6-8 hours (overnight)

Servings: 2

Ingredients

- 1 cup old-fashioned rolled oats
- 1 cup unsweetened almond milk (or milk of your choice)
- 1/2 cup fresh or frozen blueberries
- 1/4 cup plain Greek yogurt
- 2 tablespoons chia seeds
- 2 tablespoons almond butter
- 1 tablespoon honey or maple syrup (optional, for sweetness)
- 1 teaspoon vanilla extract
- 1/4 cup sliced almonds
- A pinch of salt

Procedures

Combine Ingredients: In a medium-sized bowl or two mason jars, combine the oats, almond milk, Greek yogurt, chia seeds, almond butter, honey (if using), vanilla extract, and a pinch of salt. Give everything a good stir to make sure everything is mixed evenly.

Add Blueberries: Gently fold in the blueberries. If using frozen blueberries, there's no need to thaw them; they will thaw overnight.

Refrigerate: Cover the bowl with plastic wrap or place lids on the mason jars. Refrigerate for at least 6-8 hours or overnight to allow the oats and chia seeds to absorb the liquid and soften.

Serve: In the morning, give the mixture a good stir. If the oats are too thick, add a splash of almond milk to reach your desired consistency. Top with sliced almonds for added crunch and additional blueberries if desired.

Nutritional Values (per serving)

Calories: 350

Protein: 12g

Carbohydrates: 50g

Fiber: 10g

Sugars: 12g

Fat: 12g

Saturated Fat: 1g

Sodium: 100mg

Potassium: 450mg

Calcium: 200mg

Iron: 2mg

Cooking Tips

Customizable Sweetness: Adjust the sweetness by adding more or less honey or maple syrup according to your preference. For a lower-sugar option, use a natural sweetener like stevia.

Texture Preferences: If you prefer a smoother texture, blend the almond butter into the almond milk before mixing with the oats.

Add-Ins: Feel free to add other nutritious ingredients such as flaxseeds, hemp seeds, or a scoop of protein powder for an extra boost.

Storage: Overnight oats can be stored in the refrigerator for up to 3 days, making them ideal for meal prep. Just give them a good stir and add a splash of milk before serving if they become too thick.

Health Benefits

Heart Health: The oats and almonds are rich in fiber, particularly soluble fiber, which can help lower LDL cholesterol levels, reducing the risk of heart disease.

Blood Pressure Management: Blueberries are high in antioxidants and potassium, which can help regulate blood pressure and improve overall cardiovascular health.

Digestive Health: Chia seeds add a significant amount of fiber, which aids in digestion and helps maintain regular bowel movements.

Sustained Energy: The combination of complex carbohydrates from oats, healthy fats from almonds, and protein from Greek yogurt provides sustained energy release, keeping you full and satisfied throughout the morning.

Bone Health: The inclusion of almond milk and Greek yogurt contributes to your daily calcium intake, which is essential for maintaining strong bones and preventing osteoporosis.

Antioxidant-Rich: Blueberries are packed with antioxidants, which help protect your cells from damage caused by free radicals and may reduce inflammation.

By incorporating Blueberry Almond Overnight Oats into your breakfast routine, you can enjoy a delicious, nutrient-packed meal that supports your overall health and well-being while saving time in the morning.

Spinach and Feta Breakfast Wraps

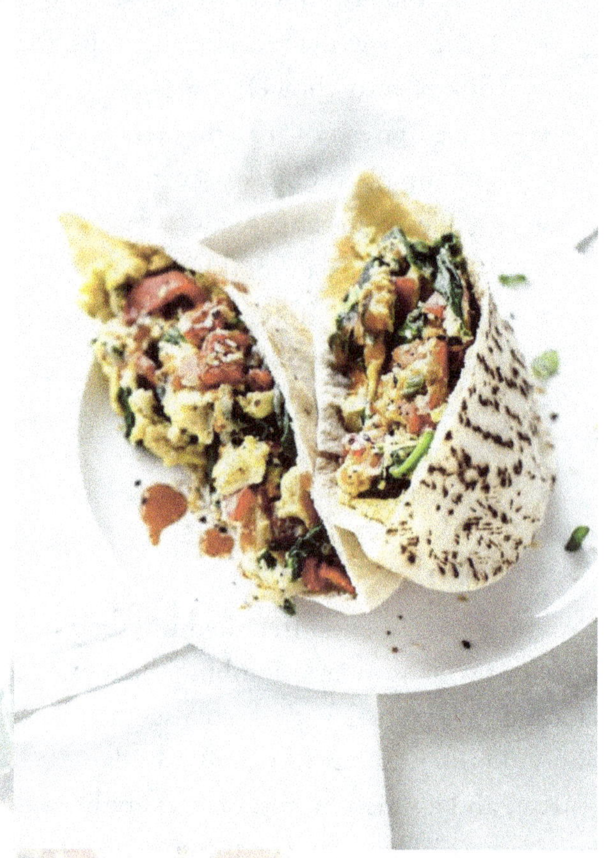

Spinach and Feta Breakfast Wraps are a delicious, nutritious way to start your day. This Mediterranean-inspired dish combines the savory flavors of spinach and feta with the satisfying texture of whole wheat wraps. It's packed with protein, fiber, and essential nutrients to keep you energized and full throughout the morning. These wraps are quick to prepare and perfect for a grab-and-go breakfast.

Preparation Time and Serving Units

Preparation Time: 10 minutes

Cooking Time: 10 minutes

Servings: 2 wraps

Ingredients

- 4 large eggs (or egg whites for a lighter option)
- 1 cup fresh spinach, chopped
- 1/2 cup crumbled feta cheese
- 2 whole wheat tortillas (8-inch size)
- 1 small tomato, diced
- 1/4 cup red onion, finely chopped
- 1 clove garlic, minced
- 1 tablespoon olive oil
- Salt and pepper to taste
- Optional: 1/2 avocado, sliced

Procedures

Prepare the Vegetables: Heat the olive oil in a non-stick skillet over medium heat. Add the red onion and garlic, sautéing for 2-3 minutes until the onion is translucent.

Add Spinach: Add the chopped spinach to the skillet and cook for another 2 minutes until wilted. Remove the spinach mixture from the skillet and set aside.

Cook the Eggs: In the same skillet, whisk the eggs (or egg whites) and pour them into the skillet. Cook, stirring occasionally, until the eggs are fully set and scrambled. Season with salt and pepper.

Combine Ingredients: Add the cooked spinach mixture back into the skillet with the eggs, mixing well. Then, add the crumbled feta cheese and diced tomato, stirring gently to combine.

Assemble the Wraps: Warm the whole wheat tortillas in the microwave or a dry skillet for a few seconds to make them more pliable.

Spoon each tortilla with half of the egg mixture.

Optional Avocado: If using, place a few slices of avocado on top of the egg mixture.

Wrap and Serve: Fold in the sides of the tortillas and roll them up tightly to form wraps. Cut each wrap in half if desired and serve immediately.

Nutritional Values (per serving)

Calories: 350

Protein: 20g

Carbohydrates: 28g

Fiber: 6g

Sugars: 3g

Fat: 18g

Saturated Fat: 6g

Sodium: 600mg

Potassium: 550mg

Calcium: 200mg

Iron: 3mg

Cooking Tips

Customize the Fillings: Feel free to add other vegetables like bell peppers, mushrooms, or zucchini for extra flavor and nutrients.

Lighten It Up: For a lighter option, use egg whites or a mix of whole eggs and egg whites. You can also use low-fat feta cheese.

Make Ahead: Prepare the filling ahead of time and store it in the refrigerator. In the morning, simply warm the filling and assemble the wraps.

Storage: These wraps can be stored in the refrigerator for up to 2 days. For best results, wrap them in aluminum foil and reheat in the oven or a skillet.

Health Benefits

High in Protein: Eggs provide high-quality protein, which is essential for muscle repair and maintenance. This helps keep you full and energized throughout the morning.

Rich in Vitamins and Minerals: Spinach is a powerhouse of vitamins A, C, K, and folate, as well as iron and calcium. These nutrients promote bone health, immunological response, and general health.

Heart Health: Feta cheese contains beneficial fatty acids and antioxidants that support heart health. Using olive oil as the cooking fat also contributes to cardiovascular health.

Digestive Health: Whole wheat tortillas add fiber to the meal, which promotes healthy digestion and helps maintain stable blood sugar levels.

Low Glycemic Index: The combination of protein, healthy fats, and fiber in this wrap helps stabilize blood sugar levels, making it a suitable option for those managing diabetes or looking to avoid energy crashes.

Antioxidants: The tomatoes, spinach, and red onions are rich in antioxidants, which help combat oxidative stress and inflammation in the body.

By incorporating Spinach and Feta Breakfast Wraps into your morning routine, you can enjoy a balanced, nutrient-dense meal that supports your health goals. These wraps are not only delicious but also versatile, allowing you to customize them to suit your taste and dietary preferences.

Quinoa Breakfast Bowl with Fresh Berries

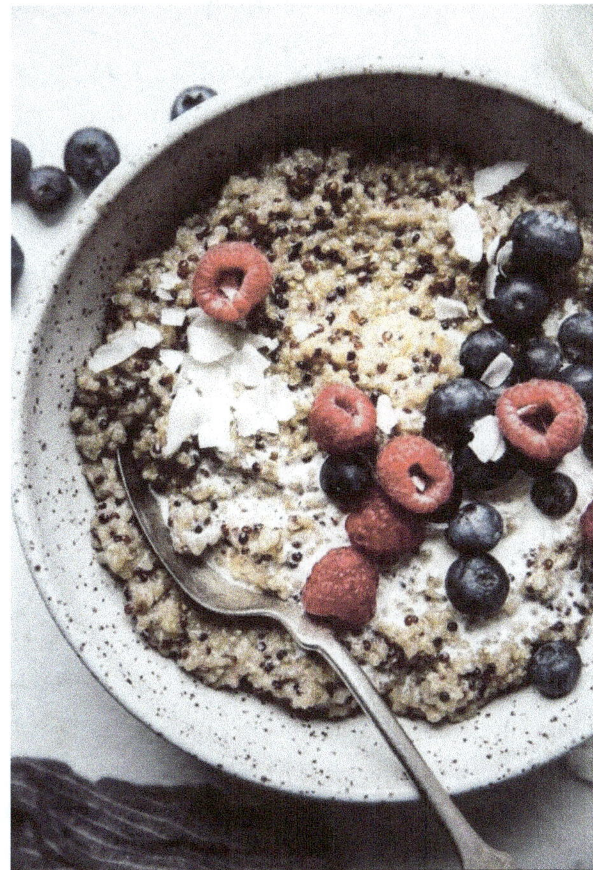

The Quinoa Breakfast Bowl with Fresh Berries is a wholesome, nutrient-dense breakfast option that combines the protein-rich qualities of quinoa with the antioxidant power of fresh berries. This bowl is perfect for a refreshing and filling start to your day. Quinoa, often regarded as a superfood, is an excellent grain alternative that provides essential amino acids, making it a complete protein source. Paired with fresh berries, nuts, and a touch of sweetness, this breakfast bowl is as delicious as it is nutritious.

Preparation Time and Serving Units

Preparation Time: 5 minutes

Cooking Time: 15 minutes

Servings: 2

Ingredients

1 cup quinoa

2 cups water

1 cup mixed fresh berries (blueberries, strawberries, raspberries, or blackberries)

1/2 cup unsweetened almond milk (or milk of your choice)

1 tablespoon honey or maple syrup

1/4 cup chopped nuts (almonds, walnuts, or pecans)

1 tablespoon chia seeds or flaxseeds

1/2 teaspoon vanilla extract

A pinch of salt

Optional toppings: sliced banana, shredded coconut, or a dollop of Greek yogurt

Procedures

Rinse Quinoa: Rinse the quinoa under cold water using a fine-mesh sieve to remove its natural coating, which can make it taste bitter.

Cook Quinoa: In a medium saucepan, combine the rinsed quinoa and water. Bring to a boil over medium-high heat. Once boiling, reduce the heat to low, cover, and simmer for about 15 minutes, or until the water is absorbed and the quinoa is tender. Take it off the heat and leave it covered for five more minutes.

Fluff and Add Flavor: Fluff the quinoa with a fork. Stir in the almond milk, honey (or maple syrup), vanilla extract, and a pinch of salt. Mix well to combine.

Prepare the Bowl: Divide the quinoa mixture into two bowls. Top each bowl with fresh berries, chopped nuts, and chia seeds (or flaxseeds).

Optional Toppings: Add any additional toppings you prefer, such as sliced banana, shredded coconut, or a dollop of Greek yogurt, for added texture and flavor.

Nutritional Values (per serving)

Calories: 350

Protein: 10g

Carbohydrates: 60g

Fiber: 10g

Sugars: 15g

Fat: 10g

Saturated Fat: 1g

Sodium: 100mg

Potassium: 400mg

Calcium: 150mg

Iron: 3mg

Cooking Tips

Batch Cooking: Cook a larger batch of quinoa and store it in the refrigerator for up to 5 days. This makes it easy to prepare breakfast bowls quickly during the week.

Fruit Variations: Use seasonal fruits to keep the bowl exciting and vary the flavors. In winter, you might opt for pomegranate seeds or citrus fruits.

Sweetness Levels: Adjust the sweetness to your preference. If you prefer a less sweet breakfast, reduce the amount of honey or maple syrup, or omit it entirely.

Milk Alternatives: Experiment with different types of milk, such as coconut milk or oat milk, to find your favorite flavor combination.

Texture and Crunch: For extra crunch, toast the nuts before adding them to the bowl. This enhances their flavor and texture.

Health Benefits

High in Protein: Quinoa is one of the few plant foods that contain all nine essential amino acids, making it a complete protein. This is crucial for muscle repair and growth.

Rich in Fiber: Both quinoa and berries are high in dietary fiber, which aids in digestion, helps maintain stable blood sugar levels, and promotes a feeling of fullness.

Antioxidant-Rich: Berries are packed with antioxidants, which help protect your cells from damage by free radicals and reduce inflammation.

Heart Health: The nuts and chia seeds add healthy fats, particularly omega-3 fatty acids, which are beneficial for heart health. Quinoa also contains heart-healthy magnesium.

Gluten-Free: This breakfast bowl is naturally gluten-free, making it suitable for individuals with gluten intolerance or celiac disease.

Low Glycemic Index: Quinoa doesn't quickly raise blood sugar levels because of its low glycemic index. This makes it a great option for those managing diabetes or looking to avoid energy crashes.

Bone Health: The inclusion of almond milk adds calcium and vitamin D to the meal, which are important for maintaining strong bones and preventing osteoporosis.

By incorporating the Quinoa Breakfast Bowl with Fresh Berries into your morning routine, you can enjoy a balanced, nutrient-packed meal that supports your overall health and well-being. This versatile breakfast option is not only easy to prepare but also adaptable to suit your taste and dietary preferences, making it a perfect choice for busy mornings.

Avocado Toast with Poached Eggs

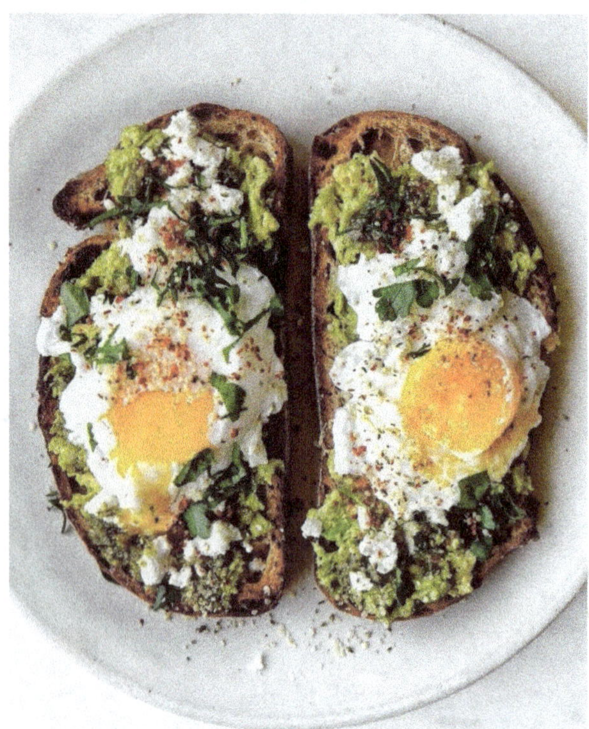

Avocado Toast with Poached Eggs is a modern breakfast classic that combines the creamy richness of ripe avocados with the protein-packed goodness of poached eggs. This dish is not only delicious but also brimming with nutrients that promote heart health, provide sustained energy, and support overall well-being. Perfect for a quick breakfast or a leisurely brunch, this recipe is both simple to prepare and versatile.

Preparation Time and Serving Units

Preparation Time: 10 minutes

Cooking Time: 10 minutes

Servings: 2

Ingredients

- 2 large eggs
- 2 slices of whole grain or sourdough bread
- 1 ripe avocado
- 1 tablespoon lemon juice
- 1 tablespoon olive oil
- Salt and pepper to taste

Optional toppings: cherry tomatoes, radishes, micro greens, red pepper flakes, feta cheese

Procedures

Prepare the Avocado: Cut the avocado in half, remove the pit, and scoop the flesh into a bowl. Add the lemon juice, pepper olive oil, and salt. Mash the avocado with a fork until it reaches your desired consistency (smooth or slightly chunky).

Toast the Bread: While preparing the avocado, toast the bread slices until they are golden brown and crispy. You can use a stovetop grill, toaster, or oven.

Poach the Eggs:

Pour water into a medium-sized saucepan and cook it gently. If desired, add a small amount of vinegar to help the eggs maintain their shape.
Crack each egg into a ramekin or small basin.

Create a gentle whirlpool in the simmering water by stirring with a spoon. Carefully slide each egg into the water. Let them cook for about 3-4 minutes, or until the whites are set but the yolks are still runny.

The poached eggs can be drained on paper towels after being taken out of the water with a slotted spoon.

Assemble the Toast: Over the toasty bread slices, equally distribute the mashed avocado. Top each piece with a poached egg.

Season and Serve: Season the eggs with a bit more salt and pepper. Add any optional toppings like cherry tomatoes, radishes, micro greens, red pepper flakes, or crumbled feta cheese for extra flavor and texture.

Nutritional Values (per serving)

Calories: 350

Protein: 12g

Carbohydrates: 28g

Fiber: 7g

Sugars: 3g

Fat: 23g

Saturated Fat: 4g

Sodium: 300mg

Potassium: 700mg

Calcium: 60mg

Iron: 2.5mg

Cooking Tips

Perfect Poached Eggs: To ensure perfectly poached eggs, use fresh eggs and maintain a gentle simmer in the water. A whirlpool can help keep the egg whites from spreading too much.

Avocado Ripeness: Choose a ripe avocado for the best texture and flavor. When squeezed, it should yield slightly under light pressure.

Bread Choice: Whole grain or sourdough bread adds a nice texture and flavor. In case you are following a strict diet, you can substitute gluten-free bread.

Variations: For added protein and flavor, consider adding smoked salmon or turkey slices beneath the poached egg.

Storage: While avocado toast is best enjoyed fresh, you can prepare the mashed avocado mixture in advance and store it in the refrigerator for up to a day. To prevent browning, cover it with plastic wrap, ensuring the wrap touches the surface of the avocado mixture.

Health Benefits

Heart Health: Monounsaturated fats, which are abundant in avocados, can help lower bad cholesterol and lower the risk of heart disease. Additionally, potassium, which helps control blood pressure, is present in them.

High in Nutrients: Avocados provide a wide range of vitamins and minerals, including vitamins K, E, C, and several B vitamins. They also contain a lot of fiber, which is good for the digestive system.

Protein-Rich: Eggs are an excellent source of high-quality protein, essential for muscle repair and maintenance. They also contain important nutrients like vitamin B12, choline, and selenium.

Sustained Energy: The combination of healthy fats from the avocado, protein from the eggs, and complex carbohydrates from the whole grain bread provides sustained energy, keeping you full and satisfied longer.

Antioxidants: Antioxidants included in avocados, such as lutein and zeaxanthin, are crucial for maintaining eye health. Eggs also provide these antioxidants, making this dish particularly beneficial for maintaining good vision.

Weight Management: This breakfast is nutrient-dense and filling, which can help control appetite and support healthy weight management.

By incorporating Avocado Toast with Poached Eggs into your breakfast routine, you can enjoy a delicious, nutrient-packed meal that supports overall health. This versatile dish is easy to customize to suit your taste preferences and dietary needs, making it a perfect choice for a balanced, energizing start to your day.

Greek Yogurt Parfait with Honey and Nuts

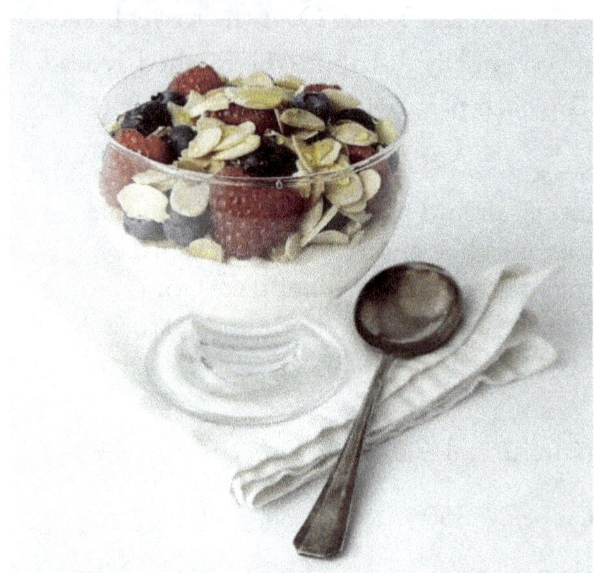

The Greek Yogurt Parfait with Honey and Nuts is a delightful and nutritious breakfast or snack option. This recipe layers creamy Greek yogurt with natural honey and a mix of crunchy nuts, creating a perfect balance of flavors and textures. Greek yogurt is rich in protein and probiotics, while honey adds a natural sweetness, and nuts contribute healthy fats and fiber. This parfait is quick to prepare, making it an ideal choice for busy mornings or a refreshing afternoon treat.

Preparation Time and Serving Units

Preparation Time: 10 minutes

Cooking Time: 0 minutes (no cooking required)

Servings: 2

Ingredients

- 2 cups plain Greek yogurt
- 2 tablespoons honey

- 1/2 cup mixed nuts (such as almonds, walnuts, pecans, and pistachios), chopped
- 1/4 cup granola (optional, for extra crunch)
- 1/2 teaspoon vanilla extract
- Fresh fruits for topping (such as berries, banana slices, or apple chunks)

Optional: for added taste, a dash of nutmeg or cinnamon

Procedures

Prepare the Nuts: Chop the mixed nuts into small pieces. You can use a variety of nuts to add different textures and flavors to the parfait.

Mix the Yogurt: In a medium bowl, combine the Greek yogurt with the vanilla extract. Stir well to evenly distribute the vanilla flavor.

Layer the Parfait: In two serving glasses or bowls, start by adding a spoonful of the Greek yogurt mixture. Drizzle a little honey over the yogurt, then sprinkle a layer of chopped nuts. If using granola, add a small amount on top of the nuts.

Repeat Layers: Continue layering with the yogurt, honey, and nuts (and granola, if using) until the glasses are full. Try to use each ingredient in at least two layers.

Add Fresh Fruits: Top the parfaits with fresh fruits of your choice. Berries, banana slices, and apple chunks are all great options that add natural sweetness and color.

Optional Spices: For an extra flavor boost, sprinkle a little cinnamon or nutmeg on top of the parfaits.

Serve Immediately: The parfaits are best served immediately to maintain the crunchiness of the nuts and granola.

Nutritional Values (per serving)

Calories: 300

Protein: 15g

Carbohydrates: 35g

Fiber: 5g

Sugars: 20g (including natural sugars from honey and fruits)

Fat: 12g

Saturated Fat: 2g

Sodium: 70mg

Potassium: 450mg

Calcium: 200mg

Iron: 2mg

Cooking Tips

Yogurt Choice: Use plain Greek yogurt for a higher protein content and a thicker texture. For a milder flavor, you can use vanilla-flavored Greek yogurt, but adjust the amount of honey accordingly.

Nut Variations: Experiment with different combinations of nuts to find your favorite mix. Toasting the nuts lightly before chopping can enhance their flavor and add an extra crunch.

Sweetness Level: To suit your taste, adjust the honey amount. If you prefer a sweeter parfait, add a bit more honey or use a flavored yogurt.

Granola Addition: For extra crunch, include a layer of granola. Choose a low-sugar granola to keep the parfait healthy.

Fruit Toppings: Seasonal fruits work best for fresh flavor. Berries are high in antioxidants, while bananas add potassium and apples provide extra fiber.

Make Ahead: Assemble the parfaits without the nuts and granola if you plan to make them ahead of time. Add the crunchy toppings just before serving to maintain their texture.

Health Benefits

High in Protein: Greek yogurt is a rich source of high-quality protein, essential for muscle repair and growth. Protein also helps keep you full and satisfied longer.

Probiotics for Gut Health: Greek yogurt contains probiotics, beneficial bacteria that support a healthy digestive system and boost the immune system.

Healthy Fats: Nuts provide healthy monounsaturated and polyunsaturated fats, which are important for heart health. These fats have the potential to cut harmful cholesterol levels and lower heart disease risk.

Natural Sweetness: Honey adds natural sweetness and contains antioxidants and antibacterial properties, making it a healthier alternative to refined sugar.

Rich in Fiber: Nuts, fruits, and granola (if used) add fiber to the parfait, which aids in digestion, helps maintain stable blood sugar levels, and promotes satiety.

Vitamins and Minerals: The combination of yogurt, nuts, and fruits provides a range of essential vitamins and minerals, including calcium, potassium, vitamin C, and iron, supporting overall health and well-being.

Antioxidant-Rich: Fresh fruits, especially berries, are rich in antioxidants, which help protect your cells from damage by free radicals and reduce inflammation.

By incorporating the Greek Yogurt Parfait with Honey and Nuts into your diet, you can enjoy a delicious, nutrient-packed meal that supports your overall health. This versatile dish is easy to customize to suit your taste preferences and dietary needs, making it a perfect choice for a quick, healthy breakfast or snack.

Lunch Recipes

Lunch is a crucial meal that provides the energy and nutrients needed to sustain you through the afternoon. In our DASH Diet Cookbook 2024, we've curated a selection of delicious, balanced lunch recipes that are both nutritious and satisfying. These recipes are designed to incorporate whole grains, lean proteins, healthy fats, and a variety of vegetables, ensuring you get a well-rounded meal that aligns with the principles of the DASH diet. Whether you're looking for quick and easy options for a busy workday or more elaborate dishes for a leisurely weekend meal, our lunch recipes cater to a variety of tastes and dietary preferences. Enjoy the benefits of eating well without compromising on flavor or convenience.

Mediterranean Chickpea Salad

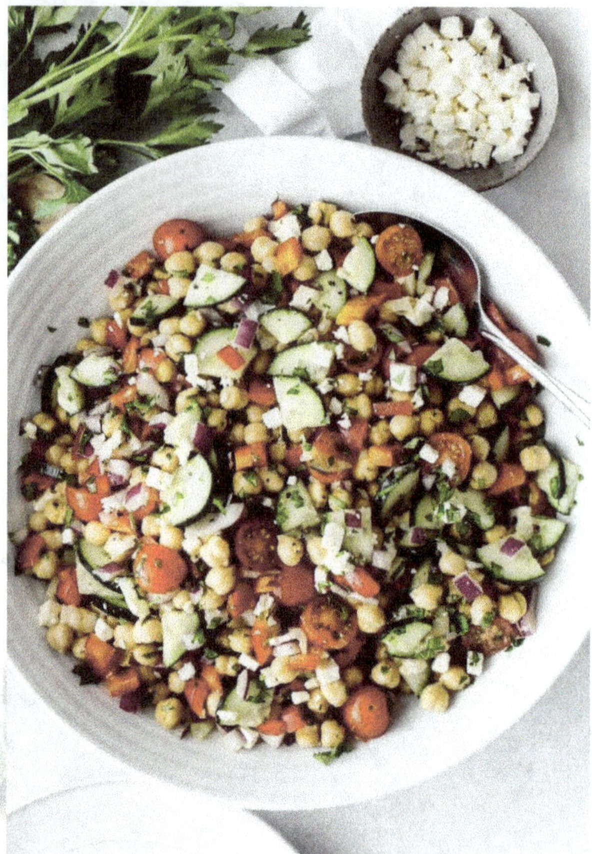

The Mediterranean Chickpea Salad is a vibrant, nutrient-rich dish that combines the flavors of the Mediterranean with the health benefits of chickpeas. This salad is packed with fresh vegetables, herbs, and a tangy lemon dressing, making it a refreshing and satisfying meal. Ideal for lunch or as a side dish, it's both easy to prepare and deliciously healthy.

Preparation Time and Serving Units

Preparation Time: 20 minutes

Cooking Time: 0 minutes (no cooking required)

Servings: 4

Ingredients

- 2 cans (15 ounces each) chickpeas, drained and rinsed
- 1 cup cherry tomatoes, halved
- 1 cucumber, diced
- 1 red bell pepper, diced
- 1/4 red onion, finely chopped
- 1/4 cup Kalamata olives, pitted and sliced
- 1/4 cup feta cheese, crumbled (optional for vegan version)
- 1/4 cup fresh parsley, chopped
- 1/4 cup fresh mint, chopped
- 1/4 cup extra-virgin olive oil
- 2 tablespoons lemon juice (freshly squeezed)
- 1 tablespoon red wine vinegar
- 1 clove garlic, minced
- Salt and pepper to taste

Optional: 1 teaspoon dried oregano or fresh oregano leaves

Procedures

Prepare the Vegetables: Start by washing and chopping all the vegetables. Halve the cherry tomatoes, dice the cucumber and red bell pepper, and finely chop the red onion.

Mix the Salad Base: In a large mixing bowl, combine the drained and rinsed chickpeas with the chopped vegetables (cherry tomatoes, cucumber, red bell pepper, and red onion).

Add the Extras: Stir in the Kalamata olives, crumbled feta cheese (if using), and fresh herbs (parsley and mint).

Make the Dressing: In a small bowl, whisk together the extra-virgin olive oil, lemon juice, red wine vinegar, minced garlic, salt, and pepper. If using, add dried oregano or fresh oregano leaves.

Combine and Toss: Pour the dressing over the chickpea mixture. Gently toss everything together until everything is fully mixed and the dressing is distributed throughout.

Adjust Seasoning: Taste the salad and adjust the seasoning with additional salt, pepper, or lemon juice as needed.

Chill and Serve: For best results, let the salad sit for at least 15 minutes before serving to allow the flavors to meld. Serve chilled or at room temperature.

Nutritional Values (per serving)

Calories: 320

Protein: 10g

Carbohydrates: 30g

Fiber: 8g

Sugars: 5g

Fat: 20g

Saturated Fat: 4g

Sodium: 400mg

Potassium: 500mg

Calcium: 100mg

Iron: 3mg

Cooking Tips

Fresh Herbs: For the most flavor, use fresh herbs. If fresh herbs are not available, dried herbs can be substituted, but use them sparingly as they have a more concentrated flavor.

Chickpeas: For a softer texture, you can lightly mash some of the chickpeas before mixing them into the salad.

Cheese Options: For a vegan version, omit the feta cheese or substitute with a plant-based cheese alternative.

Customization: Feel free to add other Mediterranean ingredients such as artichoke hearts, sun-dried tomatoes, or capers to enhance the flavor profile.

Meal Prep: This salad can be made ahead and stored in the refrigerator for up to 3 days. It's a great option for meal prep as the flavors develop even more over time.

Dressing Variations: Experiment with different dressings, such as a tahini-based dressing for a creamier texture or a balsamic vinaigrette for a sweeter taste.

Health Benefits

High in Fiber: Chickpeas are a great source of dietary fiber, which aids in digestion, helps regulate blood sugar levels, and promotes a feeling of fullness.

Rich in Plant Protein: Chickpeas provide a good amount of plant-based protein, making this salad a satisfying and nutrient-dense meal, especially for vegetarians and vegans.

Heart Health: The ingredients in this salad, such as olive oil, fresh vegetables, and chickpeas, are staples of the Mediterranean diet, which is known for its heart-protective benefits. Olive oil contains monounsaturated fats that can help lower bad cholesterol levels.

Antioxidants: Fresh vegetables like tomatoes, bell peppers, and cucumbers are rich in antioxidants, which help protect your cells from damage and reduce inflammation.

Bone Health: Feta cheese, if used, adds calcium and phosphorus, which are essential for strong bones. Chickpeas also contribute some calcium and magnesium.

Weight Management: This salad is nutrient-dense but relatively low in calories, making it a great option for those looking to manage their weight while still enjoying a flavorful and satisfying meal.

Hydration: The high water content in vegetables like cucumbers and tomatoes helps keep you hydrated.

By incorporating the Mediterranean Chickpea Salad into your lunch routine, you can enjoy a delicious, colorful, and healthful meal that supports your dietary goals. This versatile salad is not only quick and easy to prepare but also adaptable to suit various tastes and dietary needs, making it a perfect choice for a balanced and nutritious diet.

Grilled Chicken and Veggie Wraps

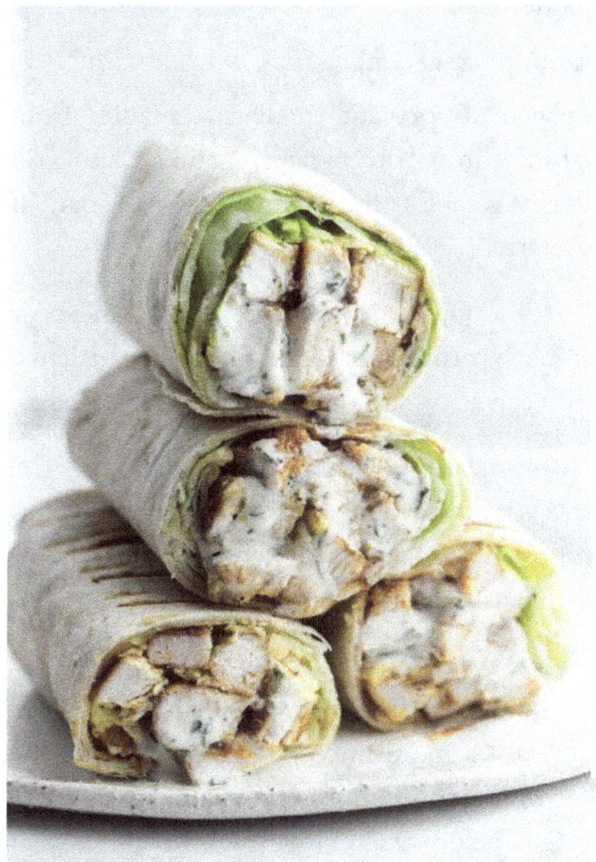

Grilled Chicken and Veggie Wraps are a flavorful and nutritious meal option that combines lean protein with an assortment of colorful vegetables, all wrapped in a soft tortilla. This dish is perfect for a quick and satisfying lunch or dinner, offering a balance of protein, fiber, vitamins, and minerals. Whether you're looking for a healthy meal on the go or a simple weeknight dinner, these wraps are sure to delight your taste buds and nourish your body.

Preparation Time and Serving Units

Preparation Time: 20 minutes

Cooking Time: 15 minutes

Servings: 4 wraps

Ingredients

- 2 boneless, skinless chicken breasts
- 4 whole wheat or spinach tortillas (10-inch size)
- 1 red bell pepper, sliced
- 1 yellow bell pepper, sliced
- 1 zucchini, sliced lengthwise
- 1 yellow squash, sliced lengthwise
- 1 red onion, sliced
- 2 tablespoons olive oil
- 1 teaspoon garlic powder
- 1 teaspoon paprika
- Salt and pepper to taste

Optional toppings: shredded lettuce, sliced avocado, hummus, Greek yogurt, feta cheese

Procedures

Preheat the Grill: Turn the heat up to medium-high on your grill.

Prepare the Chicken: Season the chicken breasts with garlic powder, paprika, salt, and pepper. Drizzle with olive oil and rub the seasonings evenly over the chicken.

Grill the Chicken: Place the seasoned chicken breasts on the preheated grill and cook for 6-8 minutes per side, or until they are cooked through and have nice grill marks. Take them off the grill and give them some time to settle before slicing.

Grill the Vegetables: While the chicken is grilling, brush the sliced bell peppers, zucchini, squash, and red onion with olive oil. Season with salt and pepper. Grill the vegetables for 3-4 minutes per side, or until they are tender and lightly charred.

Assemble the Wraps: On a level surface, arrange the tortillas. Place a few slices of grilled chicken in the center of each tortilla. Add a portion of the grilled vegetables on top of the chicken.

Optional Toppings: Add any optional toppings you like, such as shredded lettuce, sliced avocado, hummus, Greek yogurt, or crumbled feta cheese.

Wrap and Serve: Fold in the sides of the tortillas and roll them up tightly to enclose the filling. Serve each wrap right away after cutting it in half diagonally.

Nutritional Values (per wrap)

Calories: 350

Protein: 25g

Carbohydrates: 30g

Fiber: 6g

Sugars: 5g

Fat: 15g

Saturated Fat: 3g

Sodium: 450mg

Potassium: 700mg

Calcium: 100mg

Iron: 3mg

Cooking Tips

Uniform Slicing: For even cooking, try to slice the chicken breasts and vegetables to a consistent thickness.

Marinade: Marinating the chicken in your favorite marinade for at least 30 minutes before grilling can enhance its flavor and tenderness.

Grilling Vegetables: Use a grill basket or skewers to prevent smaller vegetables from falling through the grates. You can also grill the vegetables indoors on a grill pan if preferred.

Tortilla Options: Choose whole wheat or spinach tortillas for added fiber and nutrients. You can also use gluten-free tortillas if needed.

Customization: Feel free to customize the wraps with your favorite vegetables and toppings. Roasted red peppers, spinach, or thinly sliced cucumbers are all delicious additions.

Make-Ahead: Prepare the grilled chicken and vegetables in advance and store them in the refrigerator. When ready to serve, reheat them briefly before assembling the wraps.

Sauce Options: Serve the wraps with your favorite sauce or dressing on the side for dipping. Options include tzatziki, salsa, or a yogurt-based sauce with herbs.

Health Benefits

Lean Protein: Grilled chicken is a lean source of protein, essential for muscle repair and growth. Protein also helps keep you full and satisfied longer.

Vitamins and Minerals: The variety of colorful vegetables in these wraps provide essential vitamins (such as vitamin C and vitamin A) and minerals (such as potassium and magnesium) that support overall health and well-being.

Fiber-Rich: Whole wheat tortillas and vegetables are high in fiber, which aids in digestion, helps maintain stable blood sugar levels, and promotes satiety.

Heart Health: Olive oil, a staple of Mediterranean cuisine, contains monounsaturated fats that can help lower bad cholesterol levels and reduce the risk of heart disease.

Antioxidants: Bell peppers, zucchini, squash, and onions are rich in antioxidants, which help protect your cells from damage by free radicals and reduce inflammation.

Hydration: Vegetables like zucchini and squash have high water content, which helps keep you hydrated, especially during warmer months.

Versatility: These wraps are versatile and can be customized to suit various dietary preferences, including vegetarian or vegan options by omitting the chicken or adding plant-based protein alternatives.

By incorporating Grilled Chicken and Veggie Wraps into your meal rotation, you can enjoy a delicious and nutritious dish that provides a balanced combination of protein, fiber, vitamins, and minerals. These wraps are not only satisfying but also versatile, making them a perfect choice for a healthy and flavorful meal any time of the day.

Lentil and Quinoa Stuffed Peppers

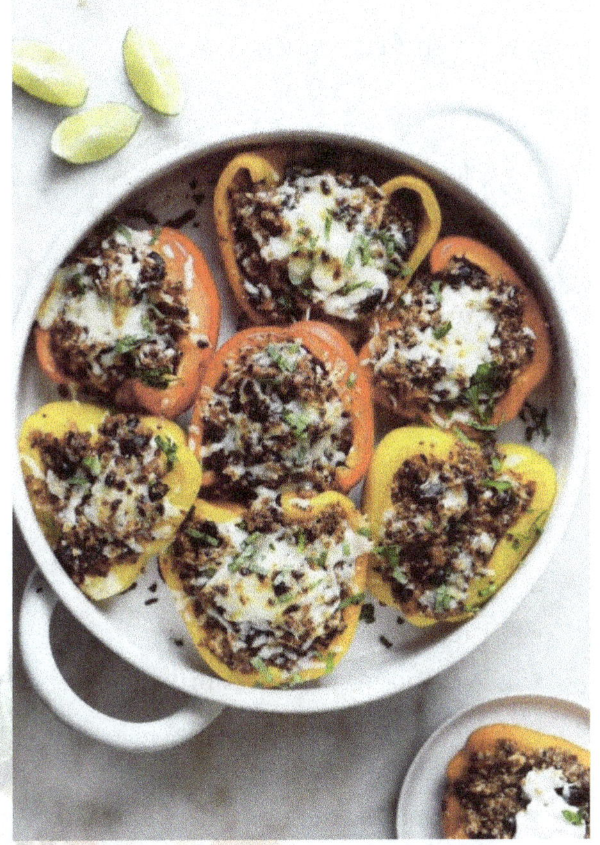

Lentil and Quinoa Stuffed Peppers are a wholesome and satisfying vegetarian dish that combines protein-rich lentils and quinoa with vibrant bell peppers, creating a nutritious and flavorful meal. These stuffed peppers are packed with fiber, vitamins, and minerals, making them a perfect choice for a healthy lunch or dinner option. Whether you're vegetarian, vegan, or simply looking to incorporate more plant-based meals into your diet, these stuffed peppers are sure to please your taste buds and nourish your body.

Preparation Time and Serving Units

Preparation Time: 20 minutes

Cooking Time: 40 minutes

Servings: 4 stuffed peppers

Ingredients

- 4 large bell peppers (any color)
- 1/2 cup uncooked quinoa, rinsed
- 1/2 cup uncooked green or brown lentils, rinsed
- 1 cup vegetable broth or water
- 1 tablespoon olive oil
- 1 onion, diced
- 2 cloves garlic, minced
- 1 carrot, diced
- 1 celery stalk, diced
- 1 teaspoon ground cumin
- 1 teaspoon smoked paprika
- 1/2 teaspoon dried thyme
- Salt and pepper to taste
- 1 can (14 ounces) diced tomatoes, drained
- 1/4 cup chopped fresh parsley or cilantro

Optional toppings: shredded cheese, avocado slices, Greek yogurt, salsa

Procedures

Preheat the Oven: Preheat your oven to 375°F (190°C). Grease a baking dish large enough to hold the stuffed peppers.

Prepare the Peppers: Cut off the bell peppers' tops to extract the seeds and membranes. Remove a small coating from the bottom of each pepper if necessary so that they stand straight in the baking dish.

Cook the Quinoa and Lentils: In a medium saucepan, combine the quinoa, lentils, and vegetable broth or water. Bring to a boil, then reduce the heat to low, cover, and simmer for 15-20 minutes, or until the quinoa and lentils are cooked and the liquid is absorbed.

Sauté the Vegetables: Heat the olive oil in a big skillet over medium heat. Add the chopped celery, carrot, onion, and garlic. Simmer the veggies for five to seven minutes, or until they are tender.

Season the Filling: Stir in the ground cumin, smoked paprika, dried thyme, salt, and pepper. To toast the spices, cook for one more minute.

Combine the Ingredients: Add the cooked quinoa and lentil mixture to the skillet with the sautéed vegetables. Stir in the diced tomatoes and chopped parsley or cilantro. Mix well to combine all the ingredients evenly.

Stuff the Peppers: Divide the quinoa and lentil mixture evenly among the hollowed-out bell peppers, pressing down gently to pack the filling.

Bake the Stuffed Peppers: Place the stuffed peppers in the prepared baking dish. Bake the casserole in a preheated oven for 25 to 30 minutes, or until the peppers are soft, covered with aluminum foil.

Optional Toppings: If desired, sprinkle shredded cheese over the stuffed peppers during the last 5 minutes of baking. Serve the stuffed peppers hot, with optional toppings such as avocado slices, Greek yogurt, or salsa.

Nutritional Values (per stuffed pepper)

Calories: 300

Protein: 12g

Carbohydrates: 50g

Fiber: 12g

Sugars: 8g

Fat: 6g

Saturated Fat: 1g

Sodium: 500mg

Potassium: 900mg

Calcium: 100mg

Iron: 4mg

Cooking Tips

Variety of Bell Peppers: Feel free to use any color of bell peppers you prefer or a combination of colors for a visually appealing presentation.

Pre-cooking Lentils and Quinoa: Ensure the lentils and quinoa are cooked before adding them to the stuffing mixture. This prevents the peppers from becoming mushy during baking.

Customization: You can customize the filling by adding other vegetables such as corn, spinach, or mushrooms, or incorporating cooked beans like black beans or kidney beans for added protein and fiber.

Spice Level: To suit your taste, vary the amount of spices. Add chili powder or cayenne pepper for extra heat if desired.

Make-Ahead Option: You can prepare the filling in advance and store it in the refrigerator for up to two days. When ready to serve, stuff the peppers and bake them as directed.

Serving Suggestions: Stuffed peppers can be served as a standalone meal or paired with a side salad or whole grain bread for a more substantial meal.

Freezing: These stuffed peppers freeze well. After baking, allow them to cool completely, then wrap them individually in plastic wrap and aluminum foil before placing them in a freezer-safe container. They can be frozen for up to three months. To reheat, thaw in the refrigerator overnight and bake in a preheated oven at 350°F (175°C) until heated through.

Health Benefits

Plant-Based Protein: Lentils and quinoa are both excellent plant-based sources of protein, providing all the essential amino acids necessary for muscle repair and growth.

High in Fiber: Lentils, quinoa, and vegetables are rich in dietary fiber, which aids in digestion, helps regulate blood sugar levels, and promotes a feeling of fullness.

Vitamins and Minerals: Bell peppers are packed with vitamins A and C, while carrots provide beta-carotene. These nutrients support immune function, vision health, and skin health.

Heart Health: The fiber, potassium, and antioxidants in this dish contribute to heart health by helping to lower blood pressure, reduce cholesterol levels, and protect against heart disease.

Weight Management: Stuffed peppers are low in calories but high in fiber and nutrients, making them a filling and satisfying option for those looking to manage their weight.

Blood Sugar Control: The complex carbohydrates in lentils and quinoa are digested slowly, leading to gradual increases in blood sugar levels and providing sustained energy throughout the day.

Digestive Health: The fiber content in this dish supports healthy digestion by promoting regular bowel movements and preventing constipation.

By incorporating Lentil and Quinoa Stuffed Peppers into your meal rotation, you can enjoy a nutritious and delicious plant-based meal that is both satisfying and wholesome. These stuffed peppers are versatile, customizable, and packed with nutrients, making them a perfect choice for anyone looking to eat healthier and enjoy the benefits of a plant-based diet.

Turkey and Avocado Spinach Salad

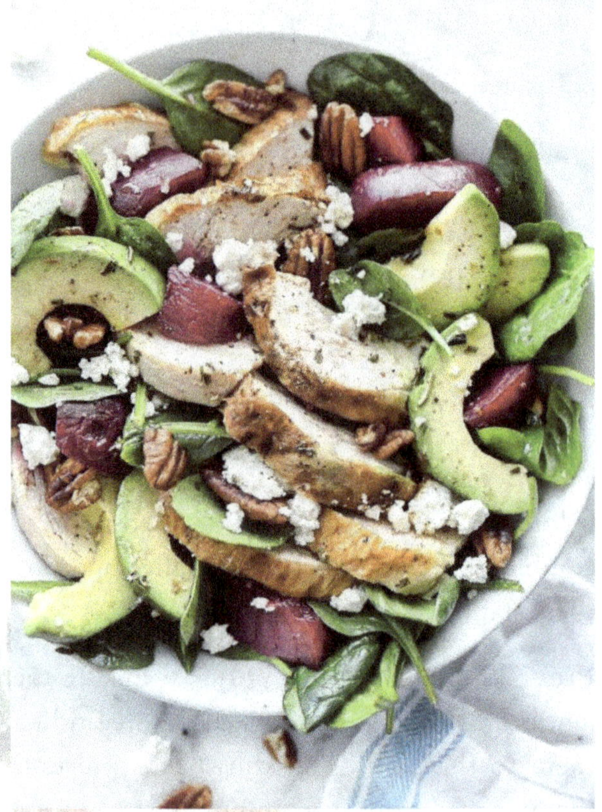

The Turkey and Avocado Spinach Salad is a delightful and nutritious dish that combines lean turkey breast with creamy avocado, fresh spinach, and a zesty vinaigrette dressing. This salad is not only delicious but also packed with protein, healthy fats, vitamins, and minerals, making it a satisfying and wholesome meal option. Whether you're looking for a light lunch, a refreshing dinner, or a healthy meal on the go, this salad is sure to satisfy your taste buds and nourish your body.

Preparation Time and Serving Units

Preparation Time: 15 minutes

Cooking Time: 10 minutes (if cooking turkey breast)

Servings: 2

Ingredients

- 2 cups fresh spinach leaves
- 1/2 lb (225g) turkey breast, cooked and sliced
- 1 ripe avocado, sliced
- 1/2 cup cherry tomatoes, halved
- 1/4 cup red onion, thinly sliced
- 1/4 cup cucumber, sliced
- 1/4 cup bell pepper, diced
- 1/4 cup crumbled feta cheese (optional)
- 2 tablespoons olive oil
- 1 tablespoon balsamic vinegar
- 1 teaspoon Dijon mustard
- Salt and pepper to taste

Optional toppings: toasted nuts or seeds, dried cranberries, sliced apple or pear

Procedures

Prepare the Salad Base: In a large mixing bowl, combine the fresh spinach leaves with the sliced turkey breast, avocado, cherry tomatoes, red onion, cucumber, and bell pepper.

Make the Dressing: Mix the olive oil, Dijon mustard, balsamic vinegar, salt, and pepper in a small bowl until thoroughly blended.

Dress the Salad: Drizzle the dressing over the salad mixture in the large bowl. Gently toss to ensure that the dressing coats every ingredient equally.

Assemble the Salad: Divide the dressed salad evenly between two serving plates or bowls.

Optional Toppings: If desired, sprinkle crumbled feta cheese over each salad portion. You can also add toasted nuts or seeds, dried cranberries, or sliced apple or pear for extra flavor and texture.

Serve Immediately: Serve the Turkey and Avocado Spinach Salad immediately, and enjoy the delicious combination of flavors and textures.

Nutritional Values (per serving)

Calories: 400

Protein: 25g

Carbohydrates: 15g

Fiber: 8g

Sugars: 4g

Fat: 28g

Saturated Fat: 5g

Sodium: 400mg

Potassium: 1000mg

Calcium: 100mg

Iron: 3mg

Cooking Tips

Cooking Turkey Breast: If using raw turkey breast, season it with your favorite herbs and spices, then grill, bake, or sauté until cooked through. Let it cool slightly before slicing.

Ripe Avocado: Choose a ripe avocado for the best flavor and texture. It should yield slightly to gentle pressure when squeezed.

Dressing Consistency: Adjust the amount of olive oil and vinegar in the dressing to achieve your desired consistency. You can also add a touch of honey or maple syrup for sweetness if desired.

Toppings Variation: Get creative with the toppings! Try adding toasted nuts or seeds for crunch, dried cranberries for sweetness, or sliced apple or pear for freshness.

Preparation Ahead: You can prepare the salad ingredients and dressing in advance and store them separately in the refrigerator. Combine them just before serving to keep the salad fresh and crisp.

Protein Alternatives: If you prefer, you can substitute the turkey breast with grilled chicken breast, shrimp, tofu, or chickpeas for a vegetarian option.

Customization: Feel free to customize the salad with your favorite vegetables, herbs, or cheese. Spinach can be substituted with mixed greens or arugula for variety.

Health Benefits

Lean Protein: Turkey breast is a lean protein source that is necessary for building and repairing muscles. Additionally, protein keeps you feeling content and full.

Healthy Fats: Monounsaturated fats found in avocados are heart-healthy and can help lower bad cholesterol and lower the risk of heart disease.

Nutrient-Dense: Spinach is rich in vitamins A, C, and K, as well as folate, iron, and potassium. These nutrients support immune function, bone health, and overall well-being.

Antioxidants: Cherry tomatoes, bell peppers, and red onions are rich in antioxidants, which help protect your cells from damage by free radicals and reduce inflammation.

Fiber-Rich: Spinach, avocado, and other vegetables in the salad are high in dietary fiber, which aids in digestion, promotes satiety, and helps regulate blood sugar levels.

Bone Health: Feta cheese (if used) adds calcium and phosphorus, which are important for maintaining strong bones and teeth.

Low-Calorie Option: This salad is relatively low in calories but high in nutrients, making it a great choice for those looking to manage their weight while still enjoying a satisfying meal.

Tomato Basil Soup with Whole Grain Bread

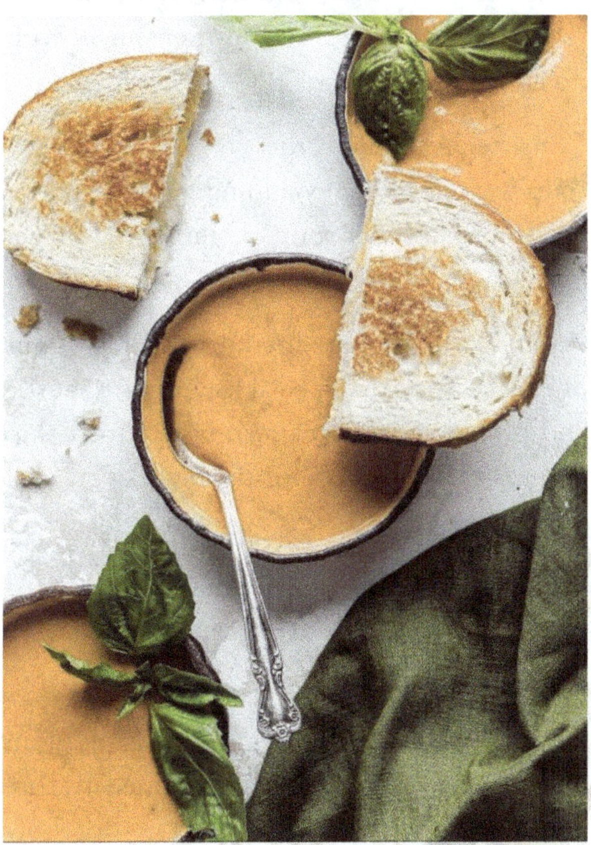

Tomato Basil Soup with Whole Grain Bread is a comforting and satisfying meal that pairs the rich flavors of tomatoes and basil with hearty whole grain bread. This classic soup is perfect for any time of year, whether you're looking for a warm and cozy meal on a chilly day or a light and refreshing option during the warmer months. Made with simple, wholesome ingredients, this soup is easy to prepare and full of nutritious goodness.

Preparation Time and Serving Units

Preparation Time: 15 minutes

Cooking Time: 30 minutes

Servings: 4

Ingredients

- 1 tablespoon olive oil
- 1 onion, chopped
- 2 cloves garlic, minced
- 2 cans (14 ounces each) diced tomatoes
- 1 can (6 ounces) tomato paste
- 4 cups vegetable broth
- 1 teaspoon dried basil
- 1/2 teaspoon dried oregano
- Salt and pepper to taste
- 1/4 cup fresh basil leaves, chopped (for garnish)
- Whole grain bread, sliced (for serving)

Procedures

Sauté the Aromatics: Heat the olive oil in a big pot or Dutch oven over medium heat. When the onion is tender, add it and sauté it for three to four minutes. Add the minced garlic and cook for an additional minute until fragrant.

Simmer the Soup: Stir in the diced tomatoes, tomato paste, vegetable broth, dried basil, dried oregano, salt, and pepper. Bring the soup to a simmer.

Cook the Soup: Reduce the heat to low and let the soup simmer for 20-25 minutes, stirring occasionally, to allow the flavors to meld together and the soup to thicken slightly.

Blend the Soup (Optional): For a smoother consistency, use an immersion blender to blend the soup directly in the pot until smooth. Alternately, pour the soup back into the pot after transferring it in batches to a blender and blending until smooth.

Adjust Seasoning: Taste the soup and adjust the seasoning with additional salt and pepper if needed.

Serve the Soup: Ladle the tomato basil soup into bowls. Garnish each serving with chopped fresh basil leaves for a burst of flavor and color.

Toast the Whole Grain Bread: While the soup is cooking, toast slices of whole grain bread until golden brown and crispy.

Serve with Bread: Serve the tomato basil soup hot, accompanied by slices of toasted whole grain bread for dipping and enjoying.

Nutritional Values (per serving, soup only)

Calories: 150

Protein: 3g

Carbohydrates: 25g

Fiber: 5g

Sugars: 10g

Fat: 5g

Saturated Fat: 1g

Sodium: 800mg

Potassium: 700mg

Calcium: 100mg

Iron: 3mg

Approximate values may differ based on certain ingredients and serving quantities.

Cooking Tips

Tomato Quality: Use high-quality canned tomatoes for the best flavor. Look for tomatoes that are packed in their juices with no added salt or sugar.

Consistency: Adjust the consistency of the soup to your liking by adding more vegetable broth for a thinner soup or simmering longer for a thicker soup.

Fresh Basil: While dried basil adds flavor during cooking, fresh basil leaves added at the end provide a vibrant, fresh taste. Don't skip the fresh basil garnish for the best flavor.

Texture Preference: If you prefer a chunkier soup, you can leave some of the diced tomatoes intact instead of blending the entire soup.

Bread Selection: Choose a hearty whole grain bread with seeds or grains for added texture and flavor. Whole grain bread is not only delicious but also provides additional fiber and nutrients.

Toasting Bread: Toasting the whole grain bread adds crunch and enhances its flavor. You can toast the bread in a toaster or under the broiler until golden brown.

Customization: Feel free to customize the soup with additional herbs and spices such as fresh thyme, rosemary, or red pepper flakes for extra heat.

Health Benefits

Rich in Lycopene: Tomatoes are rich in lycopene, a powerful antioxidant that may help reduce the risk of certain diseases, including heart disease and cancer.

Vitamins and Minerals: Tomatoes are also a good source of vitamins C, K, and potassium, as well as folate and other essential nutrients that support overall health and well-being.

Heart Health: The combination of tomatoes, olive oil, and whole grain bread provides heart-healthy fats, fiber, and antioxidants that support cardiovascular health and may help lower cholesterol levels.

Dinner Recipes

Dinner is often the heart of the day, a time to unwind and enjoy a satisfying meal. In our collection of DASH Diet Cookbook 2024 recipes, we present a variety of dinner options that are both nourishing and delicious. From hearty main courses to lighter fare, these recipes are designed to align with the principles of the DASH diet, focusing on whole foods, lean proteins, and plenty of fruits and vegetables. Whether you're cooking for one, feeding a family, or hosting guests, these dinner recipes offer something for everyone, promoting health and enjoyment around the dinner table.

Baked Salmon with Asparagus

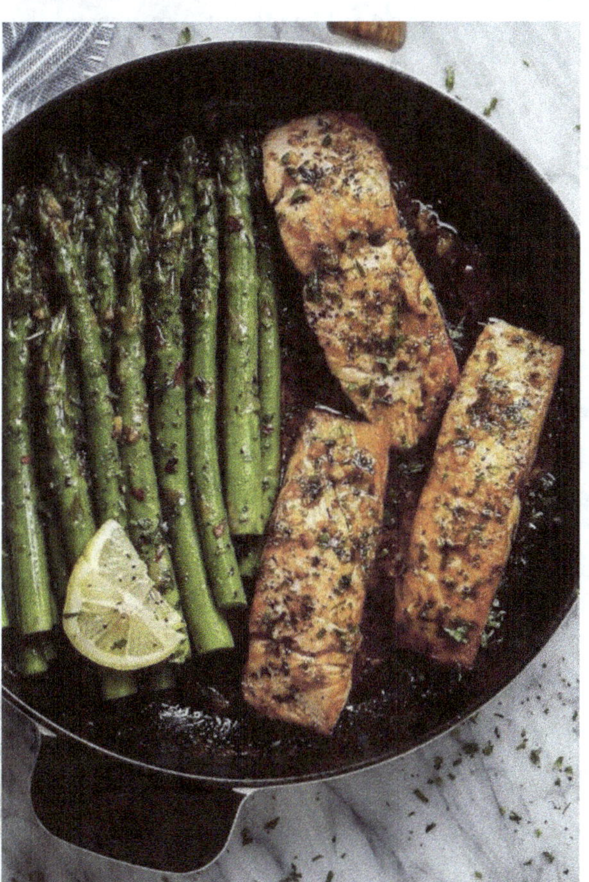

Baked Salmon with Asparagus is a simple yet elegant dish that brings together the rich flavors of salmon with the vibrant freshness of asparagus. This recipe offers a healthy and delicious way to enjoy a seafood dinner packed with omega-3 fatty acids, vitamins, and minerals. Perfect for a weeknight meal or a special occasion, this dish is sure to impress with its ease of preparation and delightful taste.

Preparation Time and Serving Units

Preparation Time: 10 minutes

Cooking Time: 20 minutes

Servings: 4

Ingredients

- 4 salmon fillets (about 6 ounces each), skin-on or skinless
- 1 bunch asparagus, trimmed
- 2 tablespoons olive oil
- 2 cloves garlic, minced
- 1 teaspoon lemon zest
- 1 tablespoon lemon juice
- 1 teaspoon dried dill (or 1 tablespoon fresh dill, chopped)
- Salt and pepper to taste
- Lemon wedges (for serving)
- Fresh dill or parsley, chopped (for garnish)

Procedures

Preheat the Oven: Set oven temperature to 400°F, or 200°C. For easier cleanup, line a baking pan with aluminum foil or parchment paper.

Prepare the Salmon: Place the salmon fillets on the prepared baking sheet, spaced slightly apart. Put the salmon skin-side down if it has any.

Prepare the Asparagus: Arrange the trimmed asparagus spears alongside the salmon fillets on the baking sheet.

Make the Seasoning: In a small bowl, whisk together the olive oil, minced garlic, lemon zest, lemon juice, dried dill, salt, and pepper to create a marinade.

Season the Salmon and Asparagus: Drizzle the marinade over the salmon fillets and asparagus, making sure to coat them evenly.

Bake the Salmon and Asparagus: Place the baking sheet in the preheated oven and bake for 15-20 minutes, or until the salmon is cooked through and flakes easily with a fork and the asparagus is tender yet still crisp.

Serve Hot: Remove the baked salmon and asparagus from the oven. Serve hot, garnished with chopped fresh dill or parsley and lemon wedges on the side.

Nutritional Values (per serving)

Calories: 300

Protein: 30g

Carbohydrates: 5g

Fiber: 2g

Sugars: 2g

Fat: 18g

Saturated Fat: 3g

Cholesterol: 80mg

Sodium: 350mg

Potassium: 800mg

Vitamin A: 20% DV

Vitamin C: 30% DV

Calcium: 6% DV

Iron: 15% DV

Cooking Tips

Salmon Selection: Choose fresh or thawed salmon fillets for the best flavor and texture. Seek for fillets with a light marine flavor that are firm to the touch.

Asparagus Preparation: Trim the tough ends of the asparagus spears before baking. You can snap off the woody ends by hand or use a knife to trim them.

Marinade Flavor: For a stronger lemon flavor, add more lemon zest and lemon juice to the marinade. You can also adjust the amount of garlic and dill to suit your taste preferences.

Even Cooking: To ensure even cooking, try to arrange the salmon fillets and asparagus spears in a single layer on the baking sheet, with some space between each piece.

Baking Time: The baking time may vary depending on the thickness of the salmon fillets. Thicker fillets may require additional baking time, while thinner fillets may cook faster.

Doneness Check: Check the salmon for doneness by inserting a fork into the thickest part of the fillet and gently twisting. The salmon should be opaque and flake readily.

Garnish: Garnish the baked salmon and asparagus with fresh herbs like dill or parsley for a pop of color and flavor. Serve with lemon wedges on the side for a bright, citrusy finish.

Health Benefits

Omega-3 Fatty Acids: Salmon is rich in omega-3 fatty acids, which are essential for heart health, brain function, and reducing inflammation in the body.

Lean Protein: Salmon is a lean source of protein, providing all the essential amino acids necessary for muscle repair and growth.

Vitamins and Minerals: Asparagus is packed with vitamins A, C, E, and K, as well as folate and potassium. These nutrients promote bone health, immunological response, and general health.

Antioxidants: Both salmon and asparagus contain antioxidants that help protect your cells from damage by free radicals and reduce inflammation in the body.

Heart Health: The combination of omega-3 fatty acids, lean protein, and vegetables in this dish supports heart health by lowering cholesterol levels, reducing blood pressure, and improving overall cardiovascular function.

Quinoa and Black Bean Stuffed Zucchini

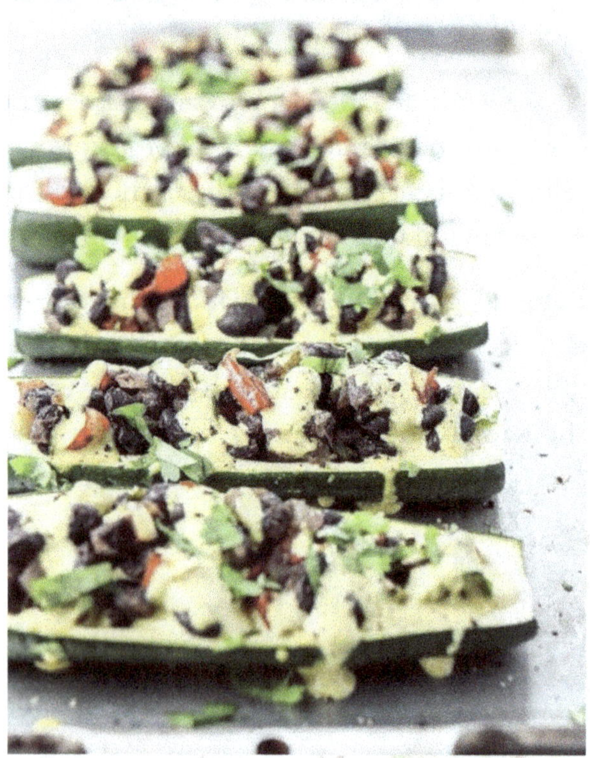

Quinoa and Black Bean Stuffed Zucchini is a nutritious and flavorful dish that combines the goodness of quinoa, protein-packed black beans, and fresh zucchini. This recipe offers a delicious way to enjoy a vegetarian meal that is both satisfying and wholesome. With a mix of hearty grains, protein-rich legumes, and vibrant vegetables, this dish is sure to become a favorite in your meal rotation.

Preparation Time and Serving Units

Preparation Time: 20 minutes

Cooking Time: 30 minutes

Servings: 4

Ingredients

- 4 medium zucchini
- 1 cup cooked quinoa
- 1 can (15 ounces) black beans, drained and rinsed
- 1 red bell pepper, diced
- 1/2 red onion, diced
- 2 cloves garlic, minced
- 1 teaspoon ground cumin
- 1 teaspoon chili powder
- Salt and pepper to taste
- 1 cup shredded cheese (cheddar, Monterey Jack, or your choice)
- Fresh cilantro or parsley, chopped (for garnish)

Optional toppings: Pieces of avocado, salsa, sour cream, or Greek yogurt

Procedures

Preheat the Oven: Preheat your oven to 375°F (190°C). Grease a baking dish large enough to hold the zucchini halves.

Prepare the Zucchini: Each zucchini should be cut in half lengthwise. Use a spoon to scoop out the flesh from the center, leaving about 1/4 inch of flesh around the edges. Keep the flesh that was scooped out for another time.

Cook the Filling: Heat the olive oil in a big skillet over medium heat. Add the minced garlic, red onion, and diced bell pepper. Sauté for 5-7 minutes, until the vegetables are softened.

Add Quinoa and Black Beans: Stir in the cooked quinoa, black beans, reserved zucchini flesh, ground cumin, chili powder, salt, and pepper. Cook for an additional 2-3 minutes to heat through and allow the flavors to meld together.

Stuff the Zucchini: Spoon the quinoa and black bean mixture into each of the hollowed-out zucchini halves, pressing down gently to pack the filling.

Top with Cheese: Sprinkle shredded cheese over the stuffed zucchini halves, covering the filling evenly.

Bake the Stuffed Zucchini: Place the stuffed zucchini halves in the prepared baking dish. Cover the dish with aluminum foil and bake in the preheated oven for 20-25 minutes, or until the zucchini is tender and the cheese is melted and bubbly.

Garnish and Serve: Take off the baking dish's foil. Garnish the stuffed zucchini with chopped fresh cilantro or parsley. Serve hot, with optional toppings such as salsa, avocado slices, Greek yogurt, or sour cream.

Nutritional Values (per serving)

Calories: 300

Protein: 15g

Carbohydrates: 35g

Fiber: 10g

Sugars: 5g

Fat: 12g

Saturated Fat: 5g

Sodium: 500mg

Potassium: 900mg

Calcium: 200mg

Iron: 4mg

Cooking Tips

Zucchini Selection: Choose medium-sized zucchini that are firm and free of blemishes. Larger zucchini may have more seeds and can be more watery.

Hollowing Zucchini: Use a spoon to hollow out the zucchini halves, being careful not to scoop out too much flesh and create holes in the bottom.

Quinoa Preparation: Cook the quinoa according to package instructions before adding it to the filling mixture. Use vegetable broth instead of water for extra flavor.

Customization: Feel free to customize the filling with your favorite vegetables or spices. Diced tomatoes, corn, spinach, or jalapeños can all be great additions.

Cheese Options: Choose your favorite type of cheese for topping the stuffed zucchini. Cheddar, Monterey Jack, pepper jack, or a Mexican blend all work well.

Baking Time: Keep an eye on the stuffed zucchini while baking to prevent overcooking. The zucchini should be tender but still hold its shape, and the cheese should be melted and golden brown.

Make-Ahead Option: You can prepare the filling mixture in advance and store it in the refrigerator for up to two days. When ready to serve, stuff the zucchini and bake as directed.

Serving Suggestions: Serve the stuffed zucchini as a main dish with a side salad or whole grain bread for a complete meal.

Leftovers can be stored in the refrigerator and reheated for a quick and easy lunch or dinner option.

Health Benefits

Plant-Based Protein: Black beans and quinoa are both excellent sources of plant-based protein, providing all the essential amino acids necessary for muscle repair and growth.

Fiber-Rich: Both black beans and quinoa are high in fiber, which aids in digestion, promotes satiety, and helps regulate blood sugar levels.

Vitamins and Minerals: Zucchini is rich in vitamins A and C, as well as potassium, which are important for immune function, vision health, and electrolyte balance.

Grilled Lemon Herb Chicken

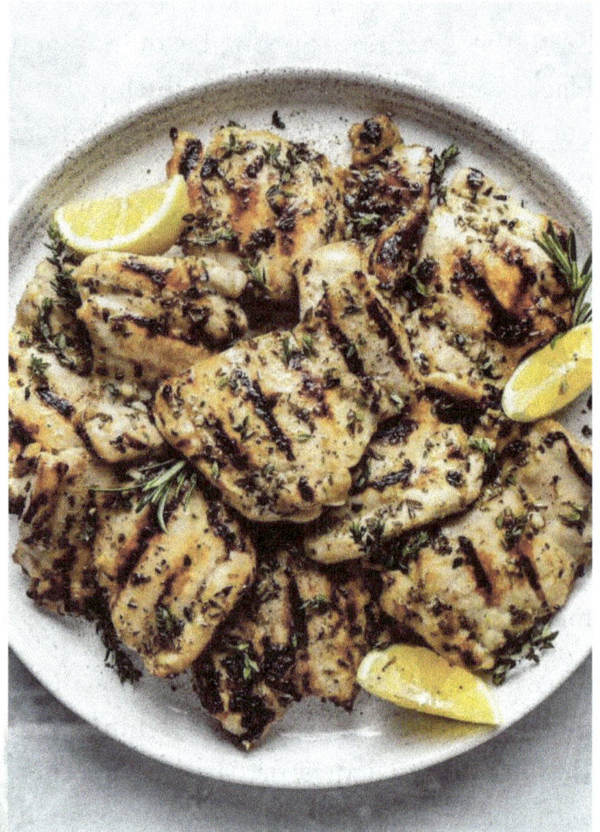

Grilled Lemon Herb Chicken is a simple yet flavorful dish that combines the zesty brightness of lemon with fragrant herbs to create a delicious and nutritious meal. This recipe is perfect for summer grilling or any time you want to enjoy tender, juicy chicken infused with fresh flavors. With minimal prep and cook time, it's a convenient option for busy weeknights or weekend gatherings with friends and family.

Preparation Time and Serving Units

Preparation Time: 10 minutes

Marinating Time: 30 minutes to 2 hours

Grilling Time: 12-15 minutes

Servings: 4

Ingredients

- 4 boneless, skinless chicken breasts
- 2 lemons, juiced and zest
- 3 cloves garlic, minced
- 2 tablespoons olive oil
- 1 tablespoon fresh parsley, chopped
- 1 tablespoon fresh thyme leaves, chopped
- 1 tablespoon fresh rosemary, chopped
- Salt and pepper to taste
- Lemon slices and fresh herbs for garnish

Procedures

Prepare the Marinade: In a small bowl, whisk together the lemon juice, lemon zest, minced garlic, olive oil, chopped parsley, thyme, rosemary, salt, and pepper to create the marinade.

Marinate the Chicken: Put the chicken breasts in a plastic bag that can be sealed or in a shallow plate. Make sure the chicken is evenly coated after pouring the marinade over it. Cover the dish or seal the bag and refrigerate for at least 30 minutes, or up to 2 hours, to allow the flavors to penetrate the meat.

Preheat the Grill: Preheat your grill to medium-high heat (about 375-400°F or 190-200°C).

Grill the Chicken: Remove the chicken from the marinade, shaking off any excess. Discard the remaining marinade. Place the chicken breasts on the preheated grill and cook for 6-8 minutes per side, or until the internal temperature reaches 165°F (75°C) and the chicken is no longer pink in the center. The thickness of the chicken breasts can affect how long they take to cook.

Rest and Serve: Once cooked through, transfer the grilled chicken to a plate and let it rest for a few minutes before serving. Garnish with lemon slices and fresh herbs for an extra burst of flavor and presentation.

Nutritional Values (per serving)

Calories: 250

Protein: 30g

Carbohydrates: 3g

Fiber: 1g

Sugars: 1g

Fat: 12g

Saturated Fat: 2g

Cholesterol: 80mg

Sodium: 300mg

Potassium: 400mg

Vitamin C: 30% DV

Iron: 6% DV

Cooking Tips

Chicken Preparation: If the chicken breasts are uneven in thickness, you can pound them to an even thickness using a meat mallet or rolling pin. This ensures even cooking.

Marinating Time: While a minimum of 30 minutes is recommended for marinating, longer marinating time (up to 2 hours) allows the flavors to penetrate deeper into the chicken, resulting in a more flavorful dish.

Grill Temperature: Make sure your grill is properly preheated to medium-high heat before adding the chicken. This helps sear the outside of the chicken quickly, sealing in juices and flavor.

Grilling Time: Avoid overcooking the chicken, as it can become dry. Check the doneness of the meat with a meat thermometer. The chicken should be cooked through to an internal temperature of 165°F (75°C).

Resting Time: Let the grilled chicken rest for a few minutes before slicing or serving. This makes the chicken juicier and more tender by allowing the juices to redistribute throughout the meat.

Fresh Herbs: For the most flavor, use fresh herbs. If you don't have fresh herbs on hand, you can use dried herbs, but use them sparingly as they are more concentrated in flavor.

Garnish: Garnish the grilled chicken with additional lemon slices and fresh herbs before serving for a beautiful presentation and extra flavor.

Health Benefits

Lean Protein: Chicken breast is a lean source of protein, which is essential for muscle repair and growth, as well as overall health and well-being.

Vitamin C: Lemon juice provides a boost of vitamin C, an antioxidant that supports immune function, collagen production, and wound healing.

Antioxidants: Fresh herbs like parsley, thyme, and rosemary are rich in antioxidants, which help protect your cells from damage by free radicals and reduce inflammation in the body.

Heart Health: Olive oil used in the marinade provides heart-healthy monounsaturated fats, which can help lower bad cholesterol levels and reduce the risk of heart disease.

Herbal Benefits: Herbs like parsley, thyme, and rosemary have been associated with various health benefits, including improved digestion, reduced inflammation, and enhanced cognitive function.

Low Carb: This grilled chicken dish is low in carbohydrates, making it suitable for low-carb or ketogenic diets.

Grilled Lemon Herb Chicken is not only delicious but also nutritious, providing a balance of protein, vitamins, and minerals in every bite. Whether you're getting ready for a summertime cookout or lighting the grill.

Vegetable Stir-Fry with Brown Rice

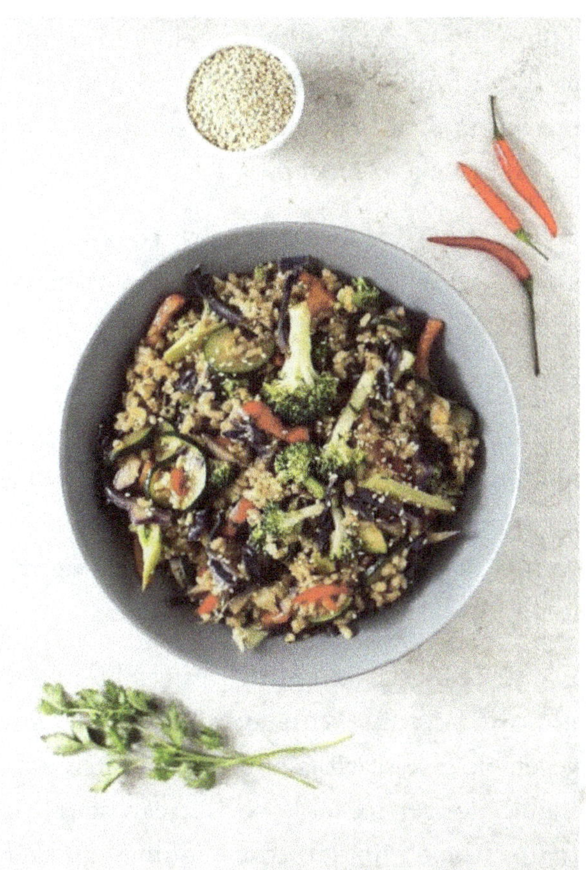

Vegetable Stir-Fry with Brown Rice is a colorful and flavorful dish that offers a perfect balance of taste and nutrition. Packed with a variety of vibrant vegetables and served with wholesome brown rice, this recipe is not only delicious but also incredibly nutritious. Stir-fries are known for their versatility, allowing you to use whatever vegetables you have on hand, making it a convenient and satisfying meal option for busy weeknights or leisurely dinners.

Preparation Time and Serving Units

Preparation Time: 15 minutes

Cooking Time: 15 minutes

Servings: 4

Ingredients

- 2 cups cooked brown rice
- 2 tablespoons vegetable oil (such as sesame oil or olive oil)
- 2 cloves garlic, minced
- 1 tablespoon fresh ginger, grated
- 1 onion, thinly sliced
- 2 cups mixed vegetables (such as bell peppers, broccoli, carrots, snap peas, mushrooms, and baby corn)
- 1 cup tofu, cubed (optional)
- 2 tablespoons soy sauce (or tamari for gluten-free option)
- 1 tablespoon rice vinegar
- 1 teaspoon sesame seeds (for garnish)
- Fresh cilantro or green onions, chopped (for garnish)

Procedures

Cook Brown Rice: If you haven't already cooked the brown rice, start by preparing it according to package instructions. Once cooked, set it aside until ready to use.

Prepare Vegetables: Wash and chop the mixed vegetables into bite-sized pieces. If using tofu, drain it well and cut it into cubes.

Heat Oil: In a large skillet or wok, heat the vegetable oil over medium-high heat.

Sauté Aromatics: Add the minced garlic and grated ginger to the hot oil and sauté for about 1 minute until fragrant.

Stir-Fry Vegetables: Add the sliced onion and mixed vegetables to the skillet. Stir-fry for 5-7 minutes, or until the vegetables are crisp-tender and slightly caramelized.

Add Tofu (Optional): If using tofu, add the cubed tofu to the skillet with the vegetables and stir-fry for an additional 2-3 minutes until heated through.

Season Stir-Fry: Drizzle soy sauce and rice vinegar over the vegetable mixture. Toss to combine, ensuring that the vegetables are evenly coated with the sauce.

Serve with Brown Rice: Divide the cooked brown rice among serving plates or bowls. Top with the vegetable stir-fry mixture.

Garnish and Serve: Garnish the vegetable stir-fry with sesame seeds and chopped cilantro or green onions for added flavor and presentation. Serve hot and enjoy!

Nutritional Values (per serving)

Calories: 300

Protein: 10g

Carbohydrates: 40g

Fiber: 6g

Sugars: 4g

Fat: 12g

Saturated Fat: 2g

Sodium: 500mg

Potassium: 600mg

Calcium: 80mg

Iron: 3mg

Cooking Tips

Vegetable Selection: Use a variety of colorful vegetables for a visually appealing stir-fry. Bell peppers, broccoli, carrots, snap peas, mushrooms, and baby corn are great options, but feel free to use any vegetables you have on hand.

Tofu Option: Tofu adds protein and texture to the stir-fry but is optional. If you're not a fan of tofu, you can omit it or substitute with cooked chicken, shrimp, or beef.

Preparation Order: Start by cooking the brown rice as it takes longer to cook than the stir-fry. While the rice is cooking, prepare and chop the vegetables and tofu.

High Heat Cooking: Stir-frying requires high heat to quickly cook the vegetables while retaining their crisp texture. Check to see if your wok or skillet is hot before adding the items.

Even Cooking: Cut the vegetables into uniform sizes to ensure even cooking. Dense vegetables like carrots and broccoli may take slightly longer to cook, so you can start stir-frying them first before adding quicker-cooking vegetables like bell peppers and snap peas.

Sauce Consistency: Adjust the amount of soy sauce and rice vinegar to suit your taste preferences. You can also add other seasonings like chili paste or sesame oil for additional flavor.

Leftovers: Leftover vegetable stir-fry can be stored in an airtight container in the refrigerator for up to 3 days. Before serving, reheat gently in the microwave or on the stovetop.

Health Benefits

Nutrient-Rich: This vegetable stir-fry is packed with vitamins, minerals, and antioxidants from the colorful array of vegetables, providing essential nutrients for overall health and well-being.

High in Fiber: Brown rice and vegetables are high in dietary fiber, which aids in digestion, promotes satiety, and helps regulate blood sugar levels.

Plant-Based Protein: Brown rice and tofu (if included) provide plant-based protein, which is important for muscle repair and growth, as well as overall health.

Low in Saturated Fat: This dish is low in saturated fat and cholesterol, making it a heart-healthy option that supports cardiovascular health.

Versatile and Customizable: Stir fries are highly versatile and can be customized based on personal preferences and dietary restrictions. You can easily adjust the ingredients and seasonings to suit your taste and nutritional needs.

Weight Management: With its balanced combination of protein, carbohydrates, and fiber, this vegetable stir-fry with brown rice can support weight management goals by providing a satisfying and nutritious meal option.

Enjoy the vibrant flavors and nutritional benefits of this Vegetable Stir-Fry with Brown Rice, a delicious and wholesome dish that's perfect for any mealtime. Whether you're cooking for yourself or sharing with family and friends, this stir-fry is sure to delight with its fresh ingredients and satisfying taste.

Beef and Broccoli Bowls

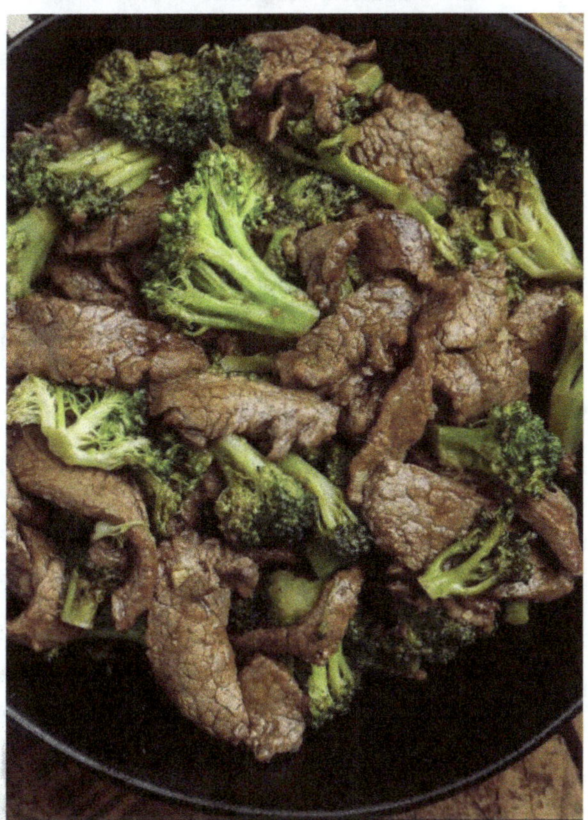

Beef and Broccoli Bowls offer a delicious and satisfying combination of tender beef, crisp broccoli, and flavorful sauce served over a bed of rice or noodles. This recipe is a crowd-pleaser, loved for its simplicity, versatility, and hearty flavors. Whether you're cooking for a weeknight dinner or preparing a special meal, these beef and broccoli bowls are sure to become a favorite in your culinary repertoire.

Preparation Time and Serving Units

Preparation Time: 15 minutes

Cooking Time: 20 minutes

Servings: 4

Ingredients

- 1 lb (450g) flank steak or sirloin, thinly sliced against the grain
- 1/4 cup soy sauce (or tamari for gluten-free option)
- 2 tablespoons oyster sauce
- 2 tablespoons brown sugar
- 2 cloves garlic, minced
- 1 teaspoon fresh ginger, grated
- 1 tablespoon cornstarch
- 2 tablespoons vegetable oil (for cooking)
- 4 cups broccoli florets
- Cooked rice or noodles, for serving
- Sesame seeds and sliced green onions, for garnish

Procedures

Marinate the Beef: In a bowl, combine the soy sauce, oyster sauce, brown sugar, minced garlic, grated ginger, and cornstarch. Make sure the beef is well coated after adding the thinly sliced steak to the marinade. Allow it to marinate in the fridge for up to an hour, or for at least 15 minutes.

Cook Rice or Noodles: While the beef is marinating, cook the rice or noodles according to package instructions. Once cooked, set aside and keep warm until ready to serve.

Sauté Broccoli: Heat a tablespoon of vegetable oil in a large skillet or wok over medium-high heat. Add the broccoli florets and stir-fry for 3-4 minutes, or until crisp-tender. After taking the broccoli out of the skillet, set it aside.

Cook Beef: In the same skillet, add another tablespoon of vegetable oil. Add the marinated beef to the skillet in a single layer, reserving any excess marinade. Cook the beef for 2-3 minutes on each side, or until browned and cooked through.

Make Sauce: While the beef is cooking, pour the reserved marinade into a small saucepan. Bring it to a simmer over medium heat and cook for 2-3 minutes, or until slightly thickened.

Combine: Once the beef is cooked, return the sautéed broccoli to the skillet. Pour the thickened sauce over the beef and broccoli, tossing to coat evenly.

Serve: Divide the cooked rice or noodles among serving bowls. Top with the beef and broccoli mixture. Add sliced green onions and sesame seeds as garnish. Serve hot and enjoy!

Nutritional Values (per serving)

Calories: 400

Protein: 25g

Carbohydrates: 35g

Fiber: 5g

Sugars: 7g

Fat: 15g

Saturated Fat: 4g

Cholesterol: 60mg

Sodium: 800mg

Potassium: 700mg

Calcium: 80mg

Iron: 3mg

Cooking Tips

Beef Selection: Choose lean cuts of beef such as flank steak or sirloin for this recipe. Slice the beef thinly against the grain to ensure tenderness.

Marinating Time: Marinating the beef adds flavor and helps tenderize the meat. If you have time, marinate the beef for at least 15 minutes, or longer for more flavor.

Vegetable Preparation: Cut the broccoli florets into bite-sized pieces for even cooking. You can also blanch the broccoli briefly in boiling water before stir-frying if you prefer a softer texture.

High Heat Cooking: Use high heat when stir-frying the broccoli and beef to achieve a nice sear and lock in flavor. Check to see if your wok or skillet is hot before adding the items.

Sauce Thickness: Adjust the thickness of the sauce to your preference by simmering it for a longer or shorter time. You can thin out the sauce with a little broth or water if it's too thick.

Garnish: Garnish the beef and broccoli bowls with sesame seeds and sliced green onions for added flavor and visual appeal. You can also drizzle with additional soy sauce or sriracha for extra seasoning.

Meal Prep: This dish is great for meal prep. You can make a big batch and store leftovers in the refrigerator for up to 3 days. Before serving, reheat gently in the microwave or on the stovetop.

Health Benefits

Protein-Rich: Beef is a good source of high-quality protein, which is essential for muscle repair and growth, as well as overall health and satiety.

Vegetable Nutrition: Broccoli is rich in vitamins, minerals, and antioxidants, including vitamin C, vitamin K, and folate, which support immune function, bone health, and cell repair.

Balanced Meal: Beef and broccoli bowls provide a balance of protein, carbohydrates, and fiber, making them a satisfying and nutritious meal option that can help maintain energy levels and support overall health.

Iron Absorption: Beef is a rich source of iron, which is important for transporting oxygen in the blood and preventing iron deficiency anemia. Pairing beef with vitamin C-rich broccoli enhances iron absorption.

Customizable: This recipe is highly customizable. You can add other vegetables such as bell peppers, carrots, or mushrooms to increase

Snacks and sides

Snacks and sides play a crucial role in rounding out a meal, offering variety, flavor, and sometimes an extra nutritional punch. From light bites to hearty accompaniments, these additions enhance the overall dining experience. In our cookbook, you'll find an array of snacks and sides ranging from crispy vegetable crudités with hummus to savory quinoa salad or roasted sweet potatoes. These options are designed to complement your main dishes while providing a satisfying and flavorful component to your meal. Whether you're looking for a quick bite to satisfy hunger between meals or a flavorful side to elevate your dish, our selection of snacks and sides has something for every palate and occasion.

Hummus and Veggie Platter

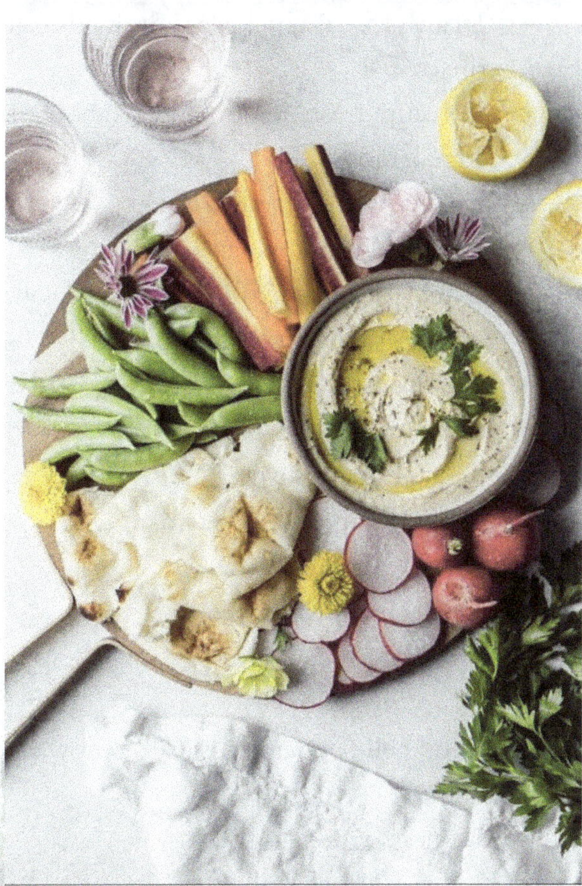

A Hummus and Veggie Platter is a delightful and nutritious option for snacking or as a side dish. It's perfect for entertaining guests, serving at parties, or enjoying as a healthy snack any time of the day. This platter features a creamy, homemade hummus paired with a variety of fresh, crunchy vegetables. It's easy to prepare, visually appealing, and packed with nutrients.

Preparation Time and Serving Units

Preparation Time: 20 minutes

Cooking Time: None

Servings: 4

Ingredients

For the Hummus:

- 1 can (15 oz) chickpeas, drained and rinsed
- 1/4 cup fresh lemon juice (about 1 large lemon)
- 1/4 cup well-stirred tahini
- 1 small garlic clove, minced
- 2 tablespoons extra-virgin olive oil, plus more for serving
- 1/2 teaspoon ground cumin
- Salt to taste
- 2-3 tablespoons water
- Dash of paprika (for garnish)
- For the Veggie Platter:
- 1 cup cherry tomatoes
- 1 cup cucumber slices
- 1 cup carrot sticks
- 1 cup bell pepper strips (red, yellow, or orange)
- 1 cup celery sticks
- 1 cup radishes, halved
- 1 cup snap peas

Procedures

Prepare the Hummus:

Blend Chickpeas and Lemon Juice: In a food processor, combine the chickpeas and lemon juice. Process for about 1 minute until creamy. If needed, scrape down the bowl's bottom and sides.

Add Tahini and Garlic: Add the tahini, minced garlic, olive oil, ground cumin, and a pinch of salt to the food processor. Process for another 30 seconds to 1 minute until well blended.

Adjust Texture: With the processor running, add 2-3 tablespoons of water, one tablespoon at a time, until the hummus reaches your desired consistency. It should be smooth and creamy.

Season to Taste: Taste the hummus and adjust the seasoning as needed, adding more salt or lemon juice if desired.

Prepare the Veggies:

Wash and Slice: Thoroughly wash all vegetables. Slice the cucumbers, carrots, bell peppers, celery, and radishes into sticks or bite-sized pieces. Halve the cherry tomatoes and trim the ends of the snap peas.

Assemble the Platter:

Arrange Veggies: On a large serving platter, arrange the sliced vegetables in groups, creating a colorful and visually appealing display.

Serve Hummus: Spoon the hummus into a serving bowl. Drizzle with a little extra-virgin olive oil and sprinkle with a dash of paprika for garnish. Place the bowl in the center of the veggie arrangement.

Serve and Enjoy: Serve the hummus and veggie platter immediately, or cover and refrigerate until ready to serve. Enjoy as a healthy snack or side dish.

Nutritional Values (per serving)

Calories: 200

Protein: 6g

Carbohydrates: 20g

Fiber: 6g

Sugars: 5g

Fat: 11g

Saturated Fat: 1.5g

Sodium: 250mg

Potassium: 500mg

Vitamin A: 100% DV

Vitamin C: 120% DV

Calcium: 6% DV

Iron: 10% DV

Cooking Tips

Hummus Variations: Customize your hummus by adding roasted red peppers, sun-dried tomatoes, or fresh herbs like parsley or cilantro. Add a dash or two of spicy sauce or a pinch of cayenne pepper for an even spicier version.

Vegetable Selection: Use a variety of colorful vegetables for a visually appealing platter. In addition to the vegetables listed, consider adding other favorites like zucchini sticks, asparagus spears, or jicama slices.

Consistency: If the hummus is too thick, add a bit more water or olive oil to achieve the desired consistency. If it's too thin, add a few more chickpeas or a bit more tahini.

Serving Suggestions: This platter pairs well with whole grain pita bread or pita chips for added variety. You can also serve it with olives, feta cheese, or pickled vegetables for a Mediterranean-inspired spread.

Storage: Store any leftover hummus in an airtight container in the refrigerator for up to 5 days. Fresh cut vegetables can also be stored in the refrigerator in a container of cold water to maintain their crispness.

Health Benefits

High in Fiber: Chickpeas and fresh vegetables are high in dietary fiber, which supports digestive health, helps maintain blood sugar levels, and promotes satiety.

Rich in Vitamins and Minerals: This platter is loaded with vitamins A, C, K, and a variety of B vitamins, as well as minerals like potassium, magnesium, and iron, which are essential for various bodily functions.

Heart-Healthy Fats: Hummus contains heart-healthy fats from tahini and olive oil, which can help reduce bad cholesterol levels and lower the risk of heart disease.

Plant-Based Protein: Chickpeas provide a good source of plant-based protein, making this a nutritious option for vegetarians and vegans.

Low Calorie and Nutrient-Dense: This dish is low in calories but nutrient-dense, making it an excellent choice for those looking to manage their weight while ensuring they get a variety of essential nutrients.

A Hummus and Veggie Platter is not only delicious and satisfying but also offers a wealth of health benefits. It's a versatile and easy-to-make dish that's perfect for any occasion, from casual snacking to elegant entertaining. Enjoy the fresh, crisp vegetables paired with creamy, flavorful hummus, and relish in the goodness of this wholesome platter.

Kale Chips with Sea Salt

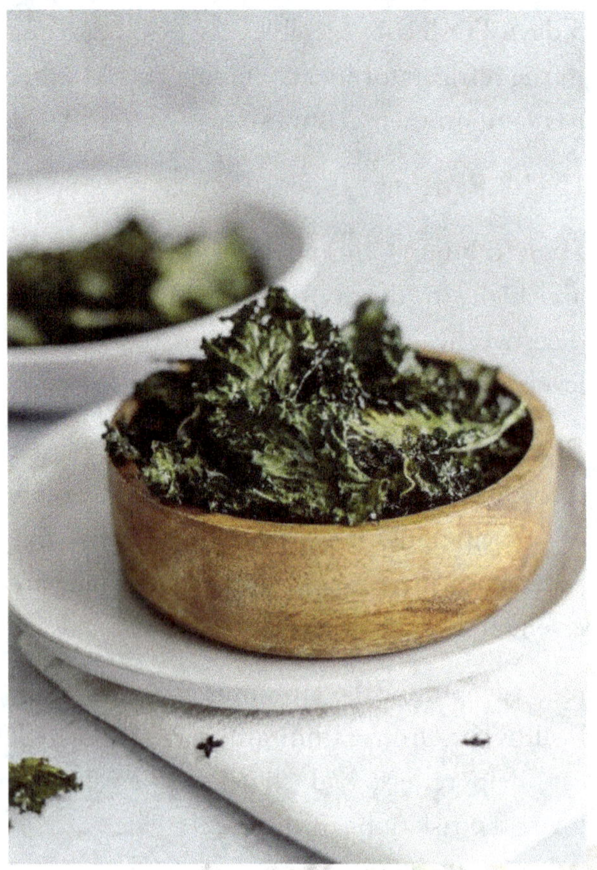

Kale Chips with Sea Salt are a crunchy, flavorful, and nutritious snack that is easy to make and perfect for satisfying your cravings for something salty and crispy. These homemade chips are made from fresh kale leaves, lightly seasoned with sea salt, and baked to perfection. They make a great alternative to traditional potato chips, providing a healthy and delicious snack option that you can enjoy anytime.

Preparation Time and Serving Units

Preparation Time: 10 minutes

Cooking Time: 20 minutes

Servings: 4

Ingredients

- 1 large bunch of kale (about 8 cups of leaves)
- 1-2 tablespoons olive oil
- 1/2 teaspoon sea salt (or to taste)

Procedures

Preheat Oven: Preheat your oven to 300°F (150°C). Use silicone baking mats or parchment paper to line a baking pan.

Prepare Kale: Wash the kale thoroughly under cold running water. Shake off the excess water and pat the leaves dry with a clean kitchen towel or paper towels. Make sure the kale is completely dry to ensure crispiness.

Remove Stems and Tear Leaves: Remove the tough stems from the kale leaves and tear the leaves into bite-sized pieces, about 2-3 inches in size.

Season Kale: Place the kale pieces in a large bowl. Add a drizzle of olive oil and a pinch of sea salt. Use your hands to massage the oil and salt evenly into the kale, ensuring all pieces are well-coated.

Arrange on Baking Sheet: Spread the seasoned kale pieces in a single layer on the prepared baking sheet. Avoid overcrowding the pan, as this will prevent the kale from becoming crispy.

Bake: Place the baking sheet in the preheated oven and bake for 20 minutes, or until the kale is crisp and lightly browned at the edges. Check the kale after 15 minutes to ensure it doesn't burn.

Cool and Serve: Remove the baking sheet from the oven and let the kale chips cool on the sheet for a few minutes. When they cool, they will keep getting crispier. Serve right away or keep for up to three days in an airtight container.

Nutritional Values (per serving)

Calories: 60

Protein: 2g

Carbohydrates: 7g

Fiber: 2g

Sugars: 0g

Fat: 3g

Saturated Fat: 0.5g

Sodium: 150mg

Potassium: 300mg

Vitamin A: 200% DV

Vitamin C: 100% DV

Calcium: 10% DV

Iron: 5% DV

Cooking Tips

Drying the Kale: Make sure the kale is completely dry before baking. Any moisture left on the leaves will cause them to steam rather than bake, resulting in soggy chips.

Even Coating: Massage the olive oil and salt into the kale thoroughly to ensure each piece is evenly coated. This helps the chips to crisp up evenly.

Single Layer: Spread the kale in a single layer on the baking sheet to allow for even cooking. Overlapping leaves will result in unevenly cooked chips.

Temperature Control: Baking at a low temperature helps to evenly dehydrate the kale without burning it. If your oven runs hot, check the chips frequently to prevent burning.

Flavor Variations: For added flavor, try sprinkling the kale with nutritional yeast for a cheesy flavor, garlic powder, smoked paprika, or chili flakes before baking.

Storage: Store any leftover kale chips in an airtight container at room temperature. If they lose their crispiness, you can re-crisp them in the oven at 300°F (150°C) for a few minutes.

Health Benefits

High in Nutrients: Kale is a nutrient-dense leafy green vegetable that provides a wealth of vitamins and minerals, including vitamins A, C, and K, as well as calcium and iron.

Rich in Antioxidants: Kale is packed with antioxidants such as beta-carotene, flavonoids, and polyphenols, which help protect the body from oxidative stress and inflammation.

Low in Calories: Kale chips are low in calories, making them a guilt-free snack option that can fit into most diet plans.

High in Fiber: The fiber content in kale aids in digestion, promotes satiety, and helps maintain healthy blood sugar levels.

Heart Health: The high levels of vitamin K and omega-3 fatty acids in kale support cardiovascular health by reducing inflammation and promoting healthy blood clotting.

Bone Health: Kale is a good source of calcium and vitamin K, both of which are important for maintaining strong and healthy bones.

Weight Management: The combination of low calories, high fiber, and high water content in kale makes it an ideal food for weight management, helping to keep you full and satisfied between meals.

Kale Chips with Sea Salt are not only a delicious and crunchy snack but also offer a variety of health benefits. Enjoy them as a standalone snack, a side dish, or a crunchy topping for salads and soups. This simple and nutritious recipe is a great way to incorporate more leafy greens into your diet in a fun and tasty way.

Sweet Potato Fries

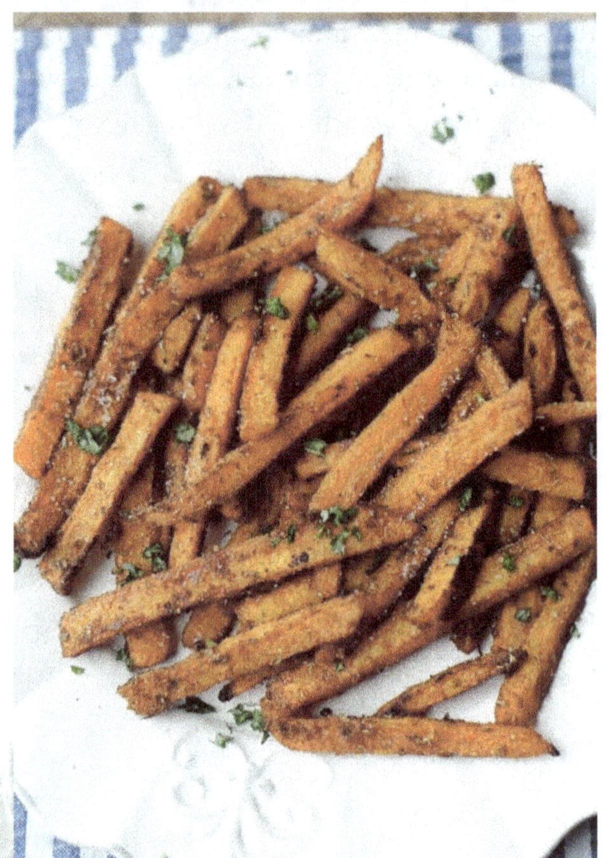

Sweet Potato Fries are a popular and healthy alternative to traditional French fries. They are deliciously crispy on the outside and tender on the inside, with a naturally sweet flavor that pairs well with a variety of seasonings. These fries are easy to make at home and can be enjoyed as a side dish, snack, or appetizer. Packed with vitamins and minerals, sweet potato fries are a nutritious addition to any meal.

Preparation Time and Serving Units

Preparation Time: 15 minutes

Cooking Time: 30 minutes

Servings: 4

Ingredients

- 2 large sweet potatoes
- 2 tablespoons olive oil
- 1 teaspoon sea salt
- 1/2 teaspoon black pepper
- 1/2 teaspoon paprika
- 1/2 teaspoon garlic powder
- 1/4 teaspoon cayenne pepper (optional, for a spicy kick)

Procedures

Preheat Oven: Preheat your oven to 425°F (220°C). Use silicone baking mats or parchment paper to line a sizable baking sheet.

Prepare Sweet Potatoes: Wash and peel the sweet potatoes. Cut them into evenly sized fries, about 1/4 to 1/2 inch thick. Try to keep the size consistent to ensure even cooking.

Season Fries: In a large bowl, toss the sweet potato fries with olive oil until they are well coated. Sprinkle with sea salt, black pepper, paprika, garlic powder, and cayenne pepper (if using). In order to spread the seasonings equally, toss again.

Arrange on Baking Sheet: Spread the seasoned sweet potato fries in a single layer on the prepared baking sheet. Make sure the fries are not overcrowded to allow for proper air circulation and even baking.

Bake: Place the baking sheet in the preheated oven and bake for 25-30 minutes, flipping the fries halfway through the baking time. Bake until the fries are golden brown and crispy on the edges.

Serve: Remove the baking sheet from the oven and let the fries cool for a few minutes. While still heated and crispy, serve right away.

Nutritional Values (per serving)

Calories: 180

Protein: 2g

Carbohydrates: 30g

Fiber: 4g

Sugars: 7g

Fat: 7g

Saturated Fat: 1g

Sodium: 400mg

Potassium: 400mg

Vitamin A: 370% DV

Vitamin C: 30% DV

Calcium: 4% DV

Iron: 6% DV

Cooking Tips

Cut Evenly: Cut the sweet potatoes into even-sized fries to ensure they cook uniformly. Thicker fries will be softer, while thinner fries will be crispier.

Avoid Overcrowding: Arrange the fries on the baking pan in a single layer. Overcrowding will cause the fries to steam rather than bake, resulting in soggy fries.

Flip Carefully: Flip the fries halfway through baking to ensure they cook evenly on all sides. Use a spatula to turn them gently.

Seasoning Variations: Experiment with different seasonings such as cinnamon and sugar for a sweet twist, or rosemary and parmesan for a savory flavor.

Dipping Sauces: Serve the sweet potato fries with a variety of dipping sauces like ketchup, aioli, or a yogurt-based dip for added flavor.

Crispier Fries: For extra crispy fries, soak the cut sweet potatoes in cold water for at least 30 minutes before seasoning. This helps remove excess starch, leading to crispier fries.

Health Benefits

Rich in Vitamins: Sweet potatoes are an excellent source of vitamin A, which is important for vision, immune function, and skin health. They also contain significant amounts of vitamin C, which supports the immune system and promotes skin health.

High in Fiber: Sweet potatoes are high in dietary fiber, which aids in digestion, helps maintain blood sugar levels, and promotes satiety, making you feel fuller for longer.

Antioxidant Properties: Sweet potatoes are rich in antioxidants like beta-carotene, which help protect the body from oxidative stress and inflammation.

Low Glycemic Index: Sweet potatoes have a lower glycemic index compared to regular potatoes, which means they have a more gradual impact on blood sugar levels, making them a better option for individuals with diabetes.

Heart Health: The high potassium content in sweet potatoes helps regulate blood pressure by counteracting the effects of sodium, thus supporting heart health.

Anti-Inflammatory: Sweet potatoes contain natural anti-inflammatory compounds that can help reduce inflammation in the body, which is beneficial for conditions like arthritis and asthma.

Sweet Potato Fries are not only a tasty and satisfying snack but also a nutritious one. They are versatile and easy to prepare, making them a great addition to any meal. Enjoy their natural sweetness and the health benefits they provide with every crispy bite.

Mixed Berry Fruit Salad

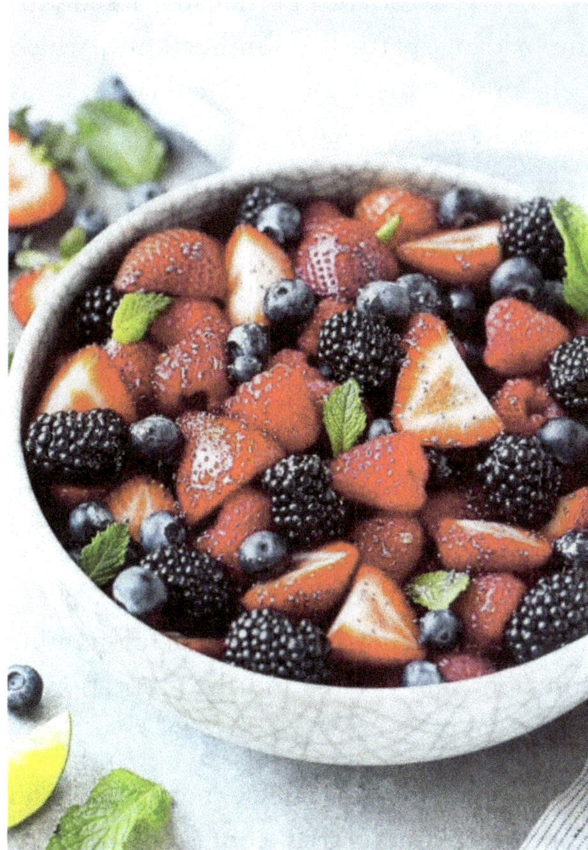

Mixed Berry Fruit Salad is a vibrant and refreshing dish that combines a variety of fresh berries, creating a colorful and nutritious treat. Perfect for breakfast, brunch, a healthy snack, or even as a dessert, this fruit salad is easy to prepare and packed with vitamins, antioxidants, and fiber. The natural sweetness of the berries requires no added sugar, making it a guilt-free indulgence that appeals to all ages.

Preparation Time and Serving Units

Preparation Time: 15 minutes

Cooking Time: None

Servings: 4

Ingredients

- 1 cup strawberries, hulled and sliced
- 1 cup blueberries
- 1 cup raspberries
- 1 cup blackberries
- 2 tablespoons fresh mint leaves, finely chopped
- 1 tablespoon fresh lemon juice
- 1 tablespoon honey (optional, for extra sweetness)

Procedures

Prepare Berries: Wash all the berries thoroughly under cold running water. Drain them well. Hull and slice the strawberries.

Combine Berries: In a large mixing bowl, gently combine the strawberries, blueberries, raspberries, and blackberries.

Add Mint and Lemon Juice: Sprinkle the chopped mint leaves over the berries. Drizzle with fresh lemon juice and honey (if using). Gently toss to combine, being careful not to crush the berries.

Chill (Optional): For best results, refrigerate the fruit salad for 15-30 minutes before serving. This facilitates the blending of flavors.

Serve: Spoon the fruit salad into a dish for serving. Garnish with a few whole mint leaves if desired, and serve immediately.

Nutritional Values (per serving)

Calories: 80

Protein: 1g

Carbohydrates: 20g

Fiber: 6g

Sugars: 12g (natural sugars from the fruit)

Fat: 0.5g

Saturated Fat: 0g

Sodium: 0mg

Potassium: 200mg

Vitamin A: 2% DV

Vitamin C: 80% DV

Calcium: 4% DV

Iron: 4% DV

Cooking Tips

Berry Selection: Choose ripe, fresh berries for the best flavor and texture. If fresh berries are not available, you can use frozen berries, but be sure to thaw and drain them thoroughly before use.

Sweetness Level: Adjust the sweetness by adding honey or a natural sweetener like agave syrup if your berries are tart. The amount can be adjusted to taste.

Mint Alternatives: If you don't have mint, fresh basil can be a delightful alternative, offering a slightly different flavor profile.

Serving Suggestions: This salad pairs wonderfully with a dollop of Greek yogurt, a sprinkle of granola, or even a scoop of vanilla ice cream for a more indulgent treat.

Storage: Any leftovers can be kept in the fridge for up to two days if they are kept in an airtight container. The berries may release some juice as they sit, so gently toss before serving.

Health Benefits

Rich in Antioxidants: Berries are packed with antioxidants, particularly anthocyanins, which help protect the body from oxidative stress and reduce inflammation.

High in Fiber: This fruit salad is high in dietary fiber, promoting healthy digestion, aiding in weight management, and helping to control blood sugar levels.

Low in Calories: With a low calorie count, this fruit salad is an excellent option for those looking to maintain or lose weight while still enjoying a satisfying treat.

Vitamin C Boost: Berries are an excellent source of vitamin C, which is vital for immune function, skin health, and the absorption of iron from plant-based foods.

Heart Health: The fiber, potassium, and antioxidants in berries contribute to heart health by lowering cholesterol levels, reducing blood pressure, and improving overall cardiovascular function.

Hydration: Berries have a high water content, which helps keep you hydrated and supports overall bodily functions.

Low Glycemic Index: Berries have a low glycemic index, meaning they have a minimal impact on blood sugar levels, making them a suitable option for individuals with diabetes.

Mixed Berry Fruit Salad is not only delicious and refreshing but also a powerhouse of nutrients. This versatile dish can be enjoyed at any time of day, offering a perfect blend of flavors and health benefits. Enjoy the natural sweetness and the burst of freshness with every bite, knowing you're nourishing your body with some of the best nature has to offer.

Roasted Garlic Brussels Sprouts

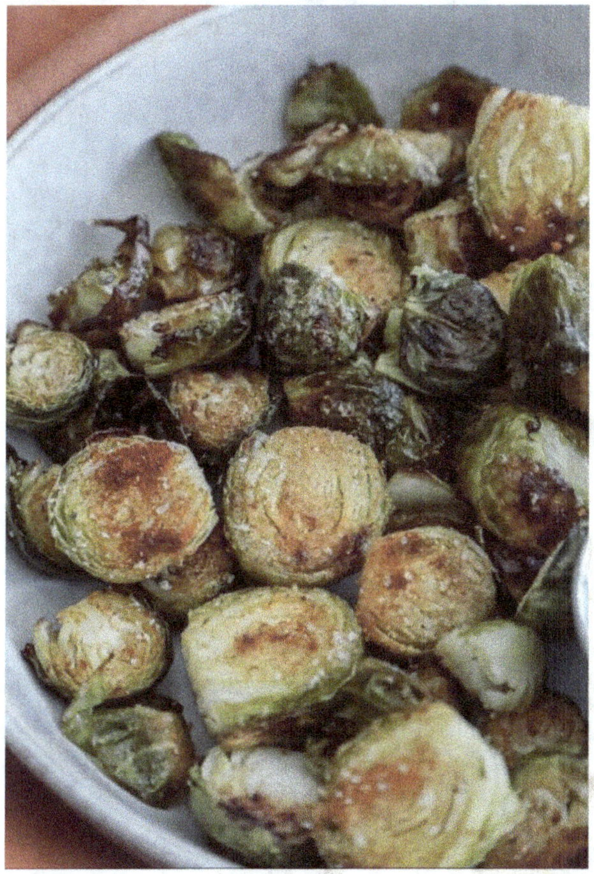

Roasted Garlic Brussels Sprouts are a delicious and nutritious side dish that complements a wide variety of main courses. Roasting brings out the natural sweetness of Brussels sprouts, while garlic adds a savory depth of flavor. This simple yet flavorful dish is easy to prepare and packed with vitamins, minerals, and antioxidants, making it a healthy addition to any meal.

Preparation Time and Serving Units

Preparation Time: 10 minutes

Cooking Time: 25-30 minutes

Servings: 4

Ingredients

- 1 pound Brussels sprouts
- 3 tablespoons olive oil
- 4 cloves garlic, minced
- 1 teaspoon sea salt
- 1/2 teaspoon black pepper
- 1 tablespoon balsamic vinegar (optional)
- 1/4 cup grated Parmesan cheese (optional)

Procedures

Preheat Oven: Preheat your oven to 400°F (200°C). A baking sheet can be lightly oiled with olive oil or lined with parchment paper.

Prepare Brussels Sprouts: Wash the Brussels sprouts thoroughly. Cut off any damaged or yellowed outer leaves, then trim the ends. Divide the Brussels sprouts lengthwise in half.

Season Brussels Sprouts: In a large mixing bowl, toss the Brussels sprouts with olive oil, minced garlic, sea salt, and black pepper until they are well coated.

Arrange on Baking Sheet: Spread the Brussels sprouts in a single layer on the prepared baking sheet. To guarantee uniform roasting, make sure they are not packed too tightly.

Roast: Place the baking sheet in the preheated oven and roast for 25-30 minutes, or until the Brussels sprouts are tender and caramelized on the edges. To guarantee even browning, stir once during the cooking process.

Add Balsamic Vinegar and Parmesan (Optional): If using, drizzle the roasted Brussels sprouts with balsamic vinegar and sprinkle with Parmesan cheese. Return to the oven for an additional 2-3 minutes to melt the cheese slightly.

Serve: Before serving, take out of the oven and allow it cool for a few minutes. Savor this as an accompaniment to your preferred main course.

Nutritional Values (per serving)

Calories: 150

Protein: 4g

Carbohydrates: 14g

Fiber: 5g

Sugars: 2g

Fat: 10g

Saturated Fat: 2g

Sodium: 300mg

Potassium: 500mg

Vitamin A: 20% DV

Vitamin C: 100% DV

Calcium: 10% DV

Iron: 8% DV

Cooking Tips

Uniform Size: Cut the Brussels sprouts to a uniform size to ensure even roasting. Smaller sprouts can be left whole, while larger ones should be halved or quartered.

Crispier Sprouts: For extra crispy Brussels sprouts, increase the oven temperature to 425°F (220°C) and roast for a slightly shorter time, checking frequently to avoid burning.

Flavor Variations: Experiment with different seasonings such as smoked paprika, chili flakes, or lemon zest for added flavor.

Avoid Overcrowding: Ensure the Brussels sprouts are spread out in a single layer on the baking sheet to promote even cooking and browning.

Garlic Timing: Add the minced garlic halfway through the roasting time if you prefer a milder garlic flavor, as garlic can burn if cooked for the full duration.

Health Benefits

High in Nutrients: Brussels sprouts are a nutrient-dense vegetable, rich in vitamins C and K, folate, and dietary fiber.

Antioxidant-Rich: These sprouts are packed with antioxidants, including kaempferol, which help protect cells from damage and reduce inflammation.

Supports Immune Health: The high vitamin C content boosts immune function and enhances skin health by promoting collagen production.

Promotes Digestive Health: Brussels sprouts are high in fiber, which aids in digestion, prevents constipation, and promotes gut health.

Bone Health: The vitamin K in Brussels sprouts is essential for bone health, aiding in bone mineralization and reducing the risk of fractures.

Cancer Prevention: Brussels sprouts contain compounds like sulforaphane, which have been shown to have cancer-fighting properties by helping to detoxify the body and protect against carcinogens.

Weight Management: Low in calories and high in fiber, Brussels sprouts can help promote feelings of fullness and aid in weight management.

Roasted Garlic Brussels Sprouts are a flavorful and nutritious side dish that can enhance any meal. Easy to prepare and versatile, this dish offers numerous health benefits while delighting your taste buds with its savory, caramelized flavors. Enjoy these roasted sprouts as a part of a balanced diet to reap their many nutritional rewards.

Dessert Recipes

essert recipes in the DASH Diet Cookbook provide a delightful and healthy way to satisfy your sweet tooth without compromising on your dietary goals. These recipes are carefully crafted to incorporate nutrient-dense ingredients, such as fruits, whole grains, and natural sweeteners, ensuring that you enjoy both flavor and nutrition. Each dessert is designed to be lower in sodium, added sugars, and unhealthy fats, while still delivering indulgent and satisfying flavors. From refreshing fruit salads to wholesome baked treats, our dessert section offers a variety of options to complement your DASH diet lifestyle. Indulge in these guilt-free desserts and enjoy a sweet ending to your healthy meals.

Dark Chocolate and Nut Clusters

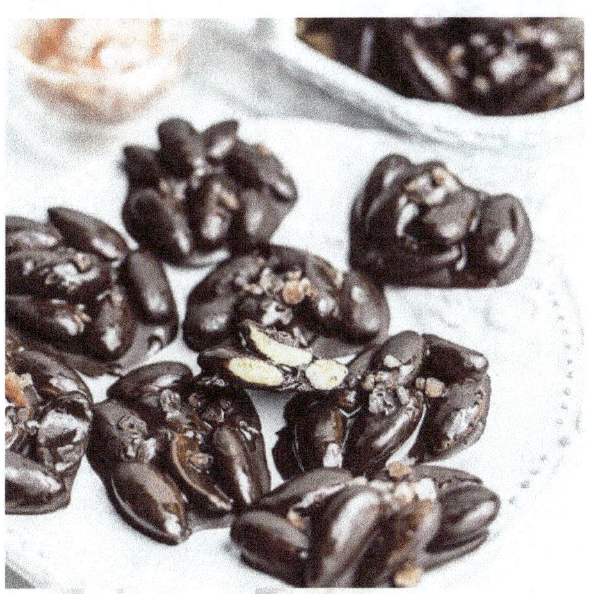

ark Chocolate and Nut Clusters are a delectable and nutritious treat that combines the rich, intense flavor of dark chocolate with the crunch and wholesome goodness of various nuts. This simple yet elegant dessert is perfect for satisfying your sweet tooth while providing essential nutrients and health benefits. Ideal for snacking, gifting, or serving as a dessert, these clusters are a healthy indulgence you can enjoy any time.

Preparation Time and Serving Units

Preparation Time: 10 minutes

Cooking Time: 5 minutes (melting chocolate)

Chilling Time: 20-30 minutes

Servings: 12 clusters

Ingredients

- 1 cup dark chocolate (70% cocoa or higher), roughly chopped
- 1/2 cup almonds, raw or lightly roasted
- 1/2 cup walnuts, raw or lightly roasted
- 1/2 cup pistachios, shelled and unsalted
- 1/4 cup dried cranberries or cherries (optional)
- 1/4 teaspoon sea salt (optional)

Procedures

Prepare Nuts: If using raw nuts, you can lightly toast them in a dry skillet over medium heat for 5-7 minutes, stirring frequently, until they are fragrant and slightly golden. Let them cool completely.

Melt Chocolate: Place the chopped dark chocolate in a heatproof bowl. Set the bowl over a pot of simmering water (double boiler method), ensuring the bottom of the bowl does not touch the water. Once the chocolate is smooth and fully melted, stir it. Alternatively, you can melt the chocolate in the microwave in 30-second intervals, stirring after each interval until fully melted.

Combine Ingredients: In a large mixing bowl, combine the almonds, walnuts, pistachios, and dried cranberries (if using). Pour the melted chocolate over the nut mixture and stir until all the nuts are evenly coated with chocolate.

Form Clusters: Line a baking sheet with parchment paper or a silicone baking mat. Using a spoon, drop small mounds of the chocolate-nut mixture onto the prepared sheet, forming clusters.

Chill: Sprinkle a small pinch of sea salt over each cluster if desired. Place the baking sheet in the refrigerator for 20-30 minutes, or until the chocolate is set and firm.

Serve: Once the clusters are fully set, transfer them to an airtight container. Store in a cool place or refrigerate. Serve chilled or at room temperature.

Nutritional Values (per cluster)

Calories: 120

Protein: 3g

Carbohydrates: 10g

Fiber: 3g

Sugars: 6g

Fat: 8g

Saturated Fat: 2.5g

Sodium: 20mg (with sea salt)

Potassium: 150mg

Vitamin E: 4% DV

Magnesium: 6% DV

Iron: 6% DV

Cooking Tips

Chocolate Quality: Use high-quality dark chocolate with at least 70% cocoa content for the best flavor and health benefits.

Nuts Selection: Feel free to customize the nuts to your preference. Hazelnuts, pecans, or cashews can be excellent substitutes or additions.

Dried Fruit: Adding dried fruits like cranberries, cherries, or apricots can enhance the clusters with a sweet-tart flavor and chewy texture. Ensure the dried fruits are unsweetened to keep the sugar content low.

Uniform Clusters: Use a small cookie scoop or spoon to form uniform clusters, ensuring even sizes for consistent serving portions.

Storage: Store the clusters in an airtight container in a cool, dry place for up to a week. For longer storage, keep them in the refrigerator for up to two weeks.

Health Benefits

Rich in Antioxidants: Dark chocolate is packed with antioxidants, particularly flavonoids, which help protect the body from oxidative stress and reduce inflammation.

Heart Health: The combination of dark chocolate and nuts can promote heart health. Dark chocolate helps improve blood flow and lower blood pressure, while nuts provide heart-healthy fats that can lower cholesterol levels.

Nutrient-Dense: Nuts are nutrient powerhouses, providing essential vitamins and minerals such as vitamin E, magnesium, and potassium, which support various bodily functions and overall health.

Weight Management: Despite being energy-dense, nuts are filling and can help control appetite and reduce overall calorie intake. The fiber and protein content in nuts contribute to satiety.

Blood Sugar Control: The combination of dark chocolate and nuts has a low glycemic index, meaning it has a minimal impact on blood sugar levels, making it suitable for individuals managing diabetes.

Mood Boosting: Dark chocolate contains compounds that can enhance mood and improve brain function by boosting the production of endorphins and serotonin.

Dark Chocolate and Nut Clusters are not only a delicious treat but also a nutritious one. Enjoy these clusters as a part of a balanced diet to satisfy your sweet cravings while reaping the numerous health benefits they offer.

Chia Seed Pudding with Fresh Mango

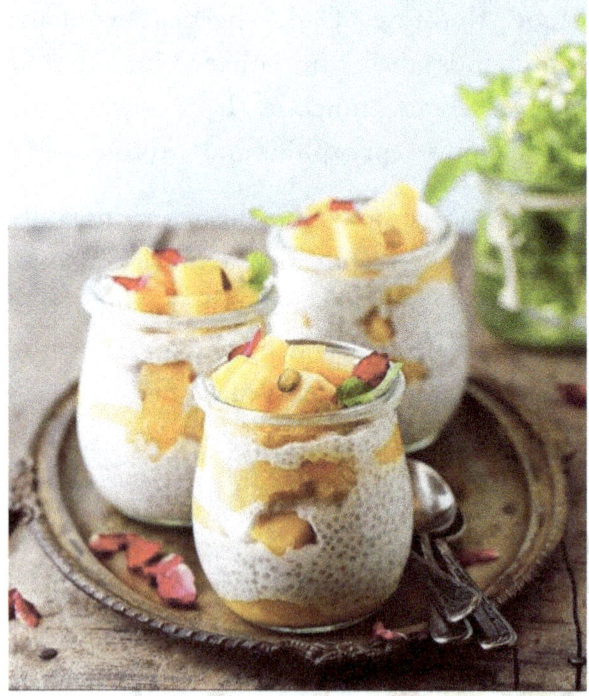

Chia Seed Pudding with Fresh Mango is a refreshing and nutritious dessert that combines the creamy texture of chia seed pudding with the sweet and tropical flavor of fresh mango. This easy-to-make, healthy treat is perfect for breakfast, snack, or dessert. Rich in omega-3 fatty acids, fiber, and vitamins, this pudding offers a delightful way to enjoy the benefits of chia seeds and fresh fruit.

Preparation Time and Serving Units

Preparation Time: 10 minutes

Cooking Time: None

Chilling Time: 4 hours (or overnight)

Servings: 4

Ingredients

- 1/2 cup chia seeds
- 2 cups unsweetened almond milk (or any plant-based milk)
- 1 tablespoon maple syrup or honey (optional)
- 1 teaspoon vanilla extract
- 2 ripe mangos, peeled, pitted, and diced
- Fresh mint leaves for garnish (optional)

Procedures

Prepare Chia Pudding: In a medium-sized mixing bowl, whisk together the chia seeds, almond milk, maple syrup (if using), and vanilla extract. Make sure the chia seeds are not clumping together and are spread evenly.

Refrigerate: Cover the bowl with plastic wrap or a lid and refrigerate for at least 4 hours, preferably overnight. This allows the chia seeds to absorb the liquid and swell, forming a pudding-like consistency.

Prepare Mango: Just before serving, peel, pit, and dice the mangos into small cubes. You can also blend one of the mangos to create a mango puree for a different texture.

Assemble the Pudding: Spoon the chia pudding into individual serving glasses or bowls. Top with a generous amount of diced mango or mango puree. If desired, garnish with fresh mint leaves.

Serve: Serve immediately for a fresh and delicious treat. The pudding can also be stored in the refrigerator for up to 2 days.

Nutritional Values (per serving)

Calories: 200

Protein: 5g

Carbohydrates: 30g

Fiber: 9g

Sugars: 18g (natural sugars from mango)

Fat: 9g

Saturated Fat: 1g

Sodium: 50mg

Potassium: 350mg

Calcium: 20% DV

Iron: 10% DV

Vitamin A: 25% DV

Vitamin C: 80% DV

Omega-3 Fatty Acids: 4500mg

Cooking Tips

Consistency: Adjust the pudding's consistency by adding more or less almond milk. If you prefer a thicker pudding, use less liquid; for a thinner consistency, add a bit more milk.

Sweetness: The natural sweetness of mango usually suffices, but you can adjust the sweetness by adding more or less maple syrup or honey according to your taste.

Flavor Variations: Experiment with different flavorings such as almond extract, coconut milk, or adding a pinch of cinnamon for a unique twist.

Fruit Alternatives: While mango pairs beautifully with chia pudding, you can substitute with other fruits like berries, kiwi, or pineapple for variety.

Blending: For a smoother texture, blend the chia seed mixture before refrigerating to break down the seeds. This creates a more uniform pudding consistency.

Health Benefits

Rich in Omega-3 Fatty Acids: Chia seeds are an excellent plant-based source of omega-3 fatty acids, which are essential for heart health and reducing inflammation.

High in Fiber: Both chia seeds and mangoes are high in dietary fiber, promoting healthy digestion, aiding in weight management, and helping to control blood sugar levels.

Nutrient-Dense: Chia seeds provide a variety of essential nutrients, including calcium, iron, and magnesium. Mangoes are rich in vitamins A and C, enhancing immune function and skin health.

Antioxidant-Rich: Mangoes contain antioxidants like quercetin and beta-carotene, which help protect the body from oxidative stress and support overall health.

Hydration: The high water content in both the chia seed pudding (due to the almond milk) and fresh mango helps keep you hydrated.

Weight Management: The combination of fiber, healthy fats, and protein in chia seeds promotes satiety, helping to reduce overall calorie intake and supporting weight management efforts.

Bone Health: Chia seeds are a good source of calcium, phosphorus, and magnesium, which are important for maintaining strong bones and preventing osteoporosis.

Chia Seed Pudding with Fresh Mango is a delicious and versatile recipe that offers numerous health benefits. Easy to prepare and customize, this pudding makes a perfect nutritious snack or dessert that you can enjoy guilt-free. Embrace the tropical flavors and creamy texture while nourishing your body with essential nutrients.

Baked Apples with Cinnamon and Walnuts

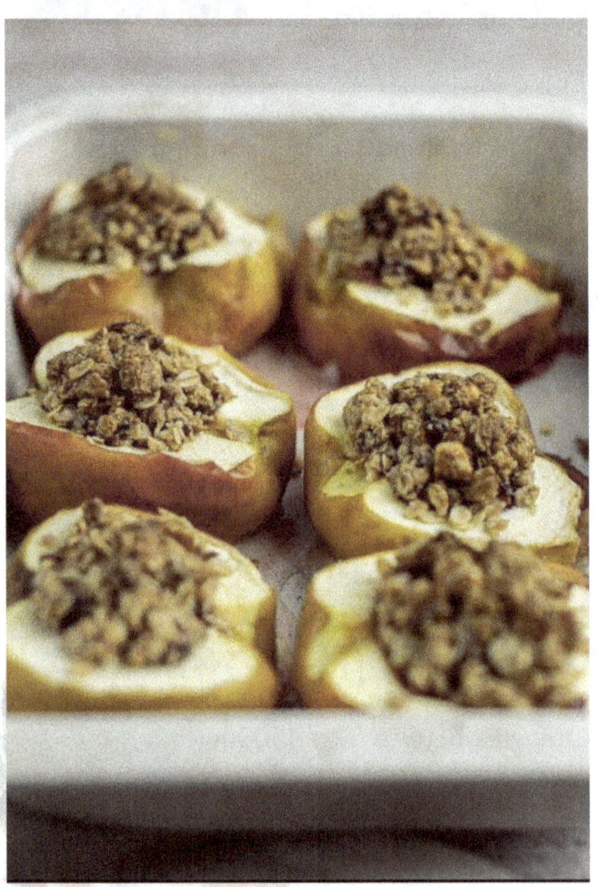

Baked Apples with Cinnamon and Walnuts is a warm and comforting dessert that brings together the natural sweetness of apples, the warm spice of cinnamon, and the rich, nutty flavor of walnuts. This simple yet delicious recipe is perfect for fall and winter evenings, offering a healthier alternative to traditional desserts. It's a treat that not only satisfies your sweet tooth but also provides numerous health benefits.

Preparation Time and Serving Units

Preparation Time: 15 minutes

Cooking Time: 35-40 minutes

Servings: 4

Ingredients

- 4 medium-sized apples (such as Granny Smith, Honey crisp, or Gala)
- 1/4 cup chopped walnuts
- 1/4 cup raisins or dried cranberries (optional)
- 1 teaspoon ground cinnamon
- 2 tablespoons honey or maple syrup
- 1 tablespoon melted butter or coconut oil
- 1 teaspoon vanilla extract
- 1/4 teaspoon ground nutmeg (optional)
- 1/2 cup water or apple juice

Procedures

Preheat Oven: Preheat your oven to 350°F (175°C).

Prepare Apples: Wash and core the apples, removing the seeds and creating a cavity about an inch wide. Take cautious not to slice through the apple all the way to the bottom.

Mix Filling: In a small bowl, combine the chopped walnuts, raisins or dried cranberries (if using), ground cinnamon, honey or maple syrup, melted butter or coconut oil, vanilla extract, and nutmeg. To guarantee that the ingredients are dispersed uniformly, thoroughly mix.

Stuff Apples: Spoon the walnut mixture into the cavities of the apples, pressing down lightly to pack the filling.

Prepare Baking Dish: Place the stuffed apples in a baking dish. Pour the water or apple juice into the bottom of the dish to help steam the apples and keep them moist during baking.

Bake: Bake the baking dish for 20 minutes in a preheated oven covered with aluminum foil. Remove the foil and continue baking for an additional 15-20 minutes, or until the apples are tender and the filling is golden and bubbly.

Serve: Allow the baked apples to cool for a few minutes before serving. Enjoy them warm, optionally with a dollop of Greek yogurt or a scoop of vanilla ice cream for an extra treat.

Nutritional Values (per serving)

Calories: 180

Protein: 1g

Carbohydrates: 35g

Fiber: 5g

Sugars: 25g (natural and added)

Fat: 7g

Saturated Fat: 1.5g

Sodium: 5mg

Potassium: 200mg

Vitamin A: 2% DV

Vitamin C: 10% DV

Calcium: 2% DV

Iron: 2% DV

Cooking Tips

Apple Selection: Choose firm apples that hold up well to baking, such as Granny Smith, Honey crisp, or Gala. Softer apples may become too mushy during baking.

Uniform Size: Try to use apples of similar size for even cooking. If the apples vary in size, they may bake unevenly.

Preventing Browning: To prevent the apples from browning after coring and before stuffing, you can brush the cut surfaces with a little lemon juice.

Filling Variations: Customize the filling with different nuts such as pecans or almonds, and experiment with various dried fruits like apricots or cherries. You can also add a tablespoon of oats for extra texture.

Liquid Choice: Using apple juice instead of water can enhance the flavor of the baked apples. For an adult twist, try using a splash of bourbon or rum in the liquid.

Health Benefits

Rich in Fiber: Apples are a great source of dietary fiber, which aids in digestion, helps maintain a healthy weight, and supports heart health by lowering cholesterol levels.

Antioxidant-Rich: Apples contain antioxidants, including quercetin, which help protect your cells from oxidative damage and may reduce the risk of chronic diseases.

Anti-Inflammatory: Cinnamon has anti-inflammatory properties and can help reduce inflammation in the body, which is beneficial for overall health and well-being.

Healthy Fats: Walnuts provide healthy omega-3 fatty acids, which are essential for heart and brain health. They also offer protein and fiber, contributing to feelings of fullness and satisfaction.

Low in Calories: Despite their sweetness and rich flavor, baked apples are relatively low in calories, making them a guilt-free dessert option.

Blood Sugar Control: The fiber in apples, along with the natural sweetness, helps in controlling blood sugar levels, making this dessert a good option for those managing diabetes.

Vitamins and Minerals: This dessert is a good source of essential vitamins and minerals such as vitamin C and potassium, which support immune function and help regulate blood pressure.

Baked Apples with Cinnamon and Walnuts are a delightful and healthful dessert that brings together the best of nature's flavors. Simple to prepare and packed with beneficial nutrients, this dish is perfect for any occasion. Enjoy the warm, spiced aroma and comforting taste while reaping the numerous health benefits of this delicious treat.

Greek Yogurt with Honey and Pistachios

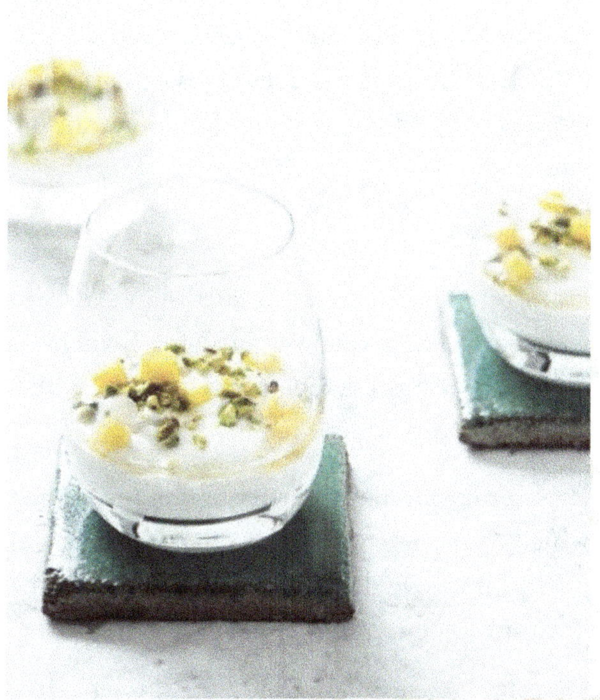

Greek Yogurt with Honey and Pistachios is a simple yet luxurious dish that combines the creamy, tangy richness of Greek yogurt with the sweetness of honey and the crunch of pistachios. This delightful recipe is perfect for breakfast, a snack, or a light dessert. It is quick to prepare, nutrient-dense, and packed with protein, healthy fats, and essential vitamins and minerals.

Preparation Time and Serving Units

Preparation Time: 5 minutes

Cooking Time: None

Servings: 4

Ingredients

- 2 cups plain Greek yogurt (full-fat or low-fat)
- 4 tablespoons honey
- 1/2 cup shelled pistachios, roughly chopped
- 1 teaspoon vanilla extract (optional)
- Fresh mint leaves for garnish (optional)
- A sprinkle of ground cinnamon (optional)

Procedures

Prepare Ingredients: Ensure the Greek yogurt is well-stirred to achieve a smooth consistency. Roughly chop the pistachios for a nice crunchy texture.

Assemble Yogurt Bowls: Divide the Greek yogurt evenly into four serving bowls.

Add Honey: Drizzle one tablespoon of honey over each bowl of yogurt. You can swirl the honey into the yogurt for an even distribution or leave it on top for a more decorative presentation.

Top with Pistachios: Sprinkle the chopped pistachios evenly over the yogurt and honey.

Optional Additions: If using, add a dash of vanilla extract to each bowl and garnish with fresh mint leaves for a burst of color and extra flavor. You can also sprinkle a pinch of ground cinnamon on top for a warm, spiced note.

Serve: Serve immediately and enjoy this delicious, nutritious treat.

Nutritional Values (per serving)

Calories: 250

Protein: 12g

Carbohydrates: 27g

Fiber: 2g

Sugars: 22g (natural sugars from honey and yogurt)

Fat: 12g

Saturated Fat: 3g

Sodium: 65mg

Potassium: 300mg

Calcium: 15% DV

Iron: 4% DV

Vitamin C: 2% DV

Vitamin A: 5% DV

Cooking Tips

Yogurt Choice: Use plain Greek yogurt to control the sweetness and flavor. Full-fat Greek yogurt provides a richer taste, while low-fat or fat-free versions are lower in calories.

Honey Variations: Experiment with different types of honey, such as wildflower, clover, or manuka, to explore varying flavor profiles.

Nut Alternatives: Substitute pistachios with other nuts like almonds, walnuts, or pecans if desired. The flavor and crunch of the almonds can be improved by toasting them beforehand.

Flavor Enhancements: Adding a touch of vanilla extract or a sprinkle of ground cinnamon can elevate the flavor of this simple dish. You can also incorporate fresh or dried fruits like berries, figs, or dates for added sweetness and texture.

Serving Suggestions: For an elegant presentation, layer the yogurt, honey, and pistachios in parfait glasses. This can also be a visually appealing option for entertaining guests.

Health Benefits

High in Protein: Greek yogurt is an excellent source of high-quality protein, which is essential for muscle repair and growth, as well as overall body function.

Probiotics: Greek yogurt contains probiotics, which are beneficial bacteria that promote gut health, improve digestion, and strengthen the immune system.

Healthy Fats: Pistachios provide healthy monounsaturated and polyunsaturated fats, which are important for heart health and reducing inflammation.

Antioxidants: Both honey and pistachios are rich in antioxidants. Honey contains phenolic compounds, and pistachios provide vitamin E and other antioxidants that help protect the body from oxidative stress.

Vitamins and Minerals: This dish is a good source of essential nutrients such as calcium, potassium, and magnesium from both the yogurt and pistachios, supporting bone health, muscle function, and overall wellness.

Low Glycemic Index: Greek yogurt and pistachios have a low glycemic index, which means they have a minimal impact on blood sugar levels. This makes this recipe a good option for those managing diabetes or looking to maintain stable blood sugar levels.

Digestive Health: The combination of protein, healthy fats, and fiber in this recipe can help promote satiety and control appetite, making it a satisfying and balanced option for various dietary needs.

Greek Yogurt with Honey and Pistachios is a versatile and nutritious recipe that is quick to prepare and full of health benefits. Whether you enjoy it for breakfast, a snack, or dessert, this delicious dish provides a perfect balance of creamy, sweet, and crunchy elements that will delight your taste buds while nourishing your body.

Strawberry Banana Smoothie

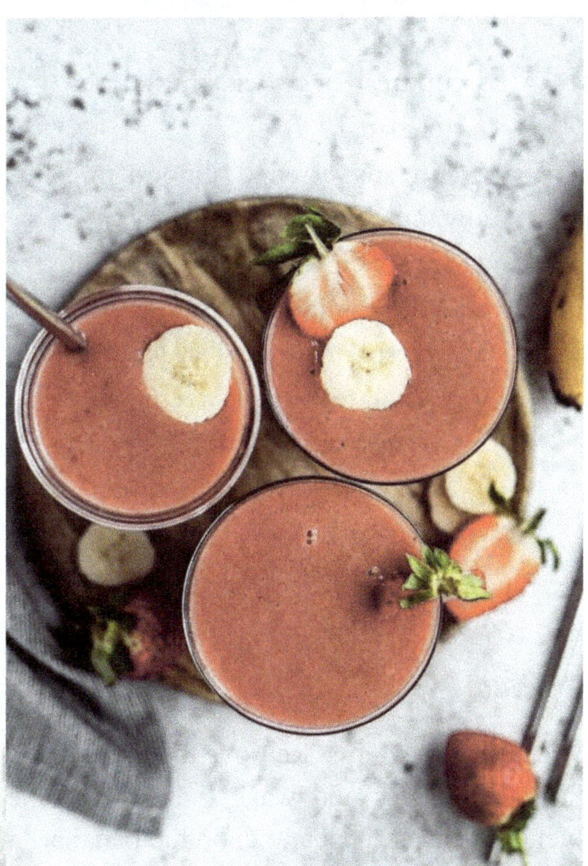

The Strawberry Banana Smoothie is a classic and refreshing beverage that combines the sweet and tangy flavors of strawberries with the creamy texture of bananas. This smoothie is perfect for a quick breakfast, a post-workout drink, or a healthy snack. It's packed with essential nutrients, including vitamins, minerals, and antioxidants, making it a delicious way to support your overall health.

Preparation Time and Serving Units

Preparation Time: 5 minutes

Cooking Time: None

Servings: 2

Ingredients

- 1 cup fresh or frozen strawberries
- 1 ripe banana
- 1 cup unsweetened almond milk (or any milk of your choice)
- 1/2 cup Greek yogurt (optional, for added creaminess and protein)
- 1 tablespoon honey or maple syrup (optional, for added sweetness)
- 1 teaspoon vanilla extract (optional)
- 1/2 cup ice cubes (if using fresh strawberries)
- Fresh mint leaves for garnish (optional)

Procedures

Prepare Ingredients: Remove the stems from the strawberries and wash them. To make blending easier, peel and chop the banana.

Blend Ingredients: In a blender, combine the strawberries, banana, almond milk, Greek yogurt (if using), honey or maple syrup (if using), and vanilla extract (if using). Add the ice cubes if you are using fresh strawberries.

Blend Until Smooth: Blend on high speed until the mixture is smooth and creamy, ensuring there are no chunks of fruit or ice remaining. This should take one to two minutes, depending on how powerful your blender is.

Serve: Pour the smoothie into two glasses. Garnish with fresh mint leaves if desired. For optimal flavor and texture, serve right away.

Nutritional Values (per serving)

Calories: 150

Protein: 5g

Carbohydrates: 30g

Fiber: 4g

Sugars: 18g (natural sugars from fruit and added sweetener)

Fat: 2g

Saturated Fat: 0g

Sodium: 60mg

Potassium: 450mg

Calcium: 20% DV

Iron: 4% DV

Vitamin C: 70% DV

Vitamin A: 2% DV

Cooking Tips

Frozen Fruit: Using frozen strawberries can give the smoothie a thicker, frostier texture. If using frozen strawberries, you may not need the ice cubes.

Sweetness Level: Adjust the sweetness by adding honey or maple syrup to taste. If the fruit is ripe and sweet, you may not need any additional sweetener.

Milk Alternatives: You can use any milk of your choice, such as dairy milk, soy milk, oat milk, or coconut milk, depending on your dietary preferences and desired flavor.

Additional Nutrients: Boost the nutritional content by adding a handful of spinach or kale for extra vitamins and minerals. The taste of the greens will be masked by the sweetness of the fruit.

Protein Boost: Add a scoop of protein powder or a tablespoon of nut butter to increase the protein content, making the smoothie more filling and suitable as a meal replacement.

Texture Variations: For a creamier smoothie, use a frozen banana. Alternatively, you can add avocado or a tablespoon of chia seeds to enhance the creaminess and nutritional profile.

Serving Suggestions: For a more substantial breakfast, serve the smoothie in a bowl and top with granola, nuts, seeds, or fresh fruit slices.

Health Benefits

Rich in Vitamins and Minerals: Strawberries and bananas are excellent sources of essential vitamins and minerals, including vitamin C, potassium, and folate, which support immune function, heart health, and overall well-being.

High in Antioxidants: Strawberries are packed with antioxidants like vitamin C and anthocyanin, which help protect your cells from oxidative stress and reduce inflammation.

Good Source of Fiber: Both strawberries and bananas provide dietary fiber, which aids in digestion, helps regulate blood sugar levels, and promotes a feeling of fullness.

Hydration: This smoothie is hydrating due to its high water content from the fruits and the almond milk, making it a refreshing choice, especially during hot weather.

Protein-Rich: Adding Greek yogurt increases the protein content, supporting muscle repair and growth, making it an excellent post-workout option.

Heart Health: The potassium in bananas and strawberries helps regulate blood pressure and supports cardiovascular health. Additionally, the antioxidants in strawberries have been linked to reduced risk of heart disease.

Weight Management: This smoothie is relatively low in calories and high in fiber and protein, helping to keep you full and satisfied, which can aid in weight management efforts.

Bone Health: Almond milk is often fortified with calcium and vitamin D, both of which are crucial for maintaining strong bones and teeth.

The Strawberry Banana Smoothie is a versatile and nutritious drink that can be tailored to fit various dietary needs and preferences. Easy to prepare and delicious, it offers a great way to start your day, replenish after a workout, or enjoy as a healthy snack.

Dr. Julie S. Clay

Beverages

Beverages play a crucial role in a balanced diet, offering hydration, essential nutrients, and a burst of flavor to complement your meals. In this section, we explore a variety of drinks that align with the DASH diet principles, emphasizing low sodium, low added sugars, and high nutrient density. From revitalizing smoothies and fruit-infused waters to herbal teas and nutrient-packed shakes, these beverage recipes are designed to not only quench your thirst but also support your overall health and well-being. Whether you need an energy boost in the morning, a refreshing drink during the day, or a calming beverage in the evening, you'll find a delicious and healthy option here.

Cucumber Mint Water

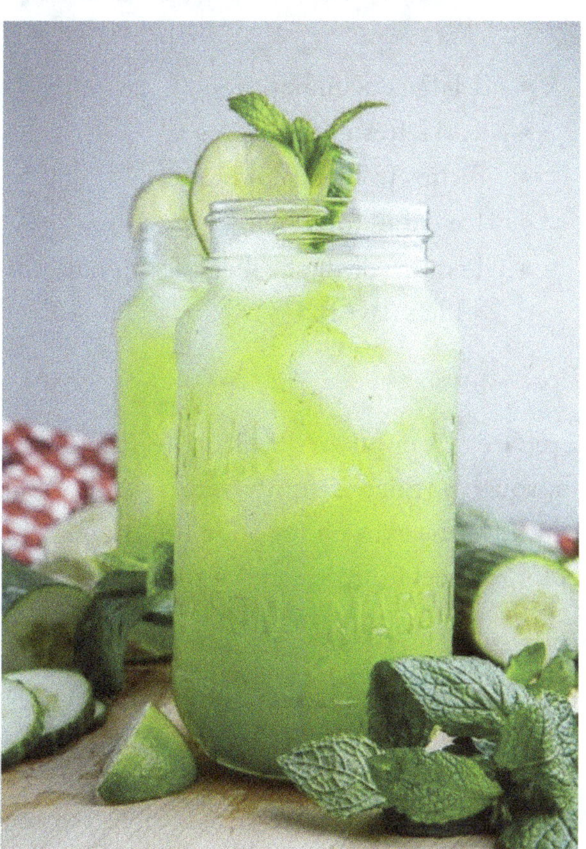

Cucumber Mint Water is a refreshing and hydrating beverage perfect for any time of the year, but especially enjoyable during warm weather. This infused water combines the crisp, cool taste of cucumbers with the invigorating flavor of fresh mint. It is a simple yet elegant way to enhance your water, making it more enjoyable to drink and helping you stay hydrated throughout the day. This drink is not only delicious but also offers various health benefits, making it an excellent addition to a healthy diet.

Preparation Time and Serving Units

Preparation Time: 10 minutes

Cooking Time: None

Servings: 8 cups (2 liters)

Ingredients

- 1 large cucumber
- 10-12 fresh mint leaves
- 8 cups (2 liters) cold water
- Ice cubes (optional)
- Lemon or lime slices (optional, for added flavor)

Procedures

Prepare Cucumber: Wash the cucumber thoroughly. Slice it thinly into rounds. You can leave the skin on for added nutrients and color, or peel it if preferred.

Prepare Mint: Rinse the mint leaves under cold water. Dry them gently with a paper towel. Lightly bruise the mint leaves by gently crushing them in your hand or using the back of a spoon. This helps to release their natural oils and flavor.

Combine Ingredients: Add the mint leaves and cucumber slices to a big pitcher. Pour in the cold water.

Infuse: Let the water sit in the refrigerator for at least 1-2 hours to allow the flavors to meld. For a stronger flavor, you can let it infuse overnight.

Serve: When ready to serve, fill glasses with ice cubes (if using) and pour the cucumber mint water over the ice. Add a few fresh cucumber slices or mint leaves for garnish if desired. For an extra twist, you can add a slice of lemon or lime to each glass.

Enjoy: Serve the water cold and enjoy its refreshing taste.

Nutritional Values (per serving, 1 cup)

Calories: 0-5

Protein: 0g

Carbohydrates: 0g

Fiber: 0g

Sugars: 0g

Fat: 0g

Saturated Fat: 0g

Sodium: 0mg

Potassium: 10mg

Vitamin C: 2% DV

Vitamin A: 1% DV

Calcium: 1% DV

Iron: 1% DV

Cooking Tips

Use Fresh Ingredients: For the best flavor, use fresh cucumbers and mint leaves. Avoid using cucumbers that are soft or have blemishes, and select mint leaves that are bright green and fragrant.

Infusion Time: The longer the water infuses, the more pronounced the flavors will be. If you prefer a milder flavor, reduce the infusion time.

Storage: Keep the infused water in the refrigerator and consume it within 24-48 hours for optimal freshness and flavor. After this period, the water may start to taste bitter or lose its refreshing quality.

Variations: Experiment with additional ingredients like lemon slices, lime slices, or a few slices of fresh ginger for a different flavor profile. You can also add a handful of berries for a hint of sweetness and extra antioxidants.

Straining: If you prefer a clearer water, you can strain the cucumber slices and mint leaves out before serving. However, leaving them in adds visual appeal and allows the flavors to continue developing.

Health Benefits

Hydration: Cucumber Mint Water is an excellent way to stay hydrated, especially for those who find plain water boring. Proper hydration is essential for maintaining bodily functions, regulating temperature, and supporting overall health.

Low-Calorie: This beverage is virtually calorie-free, making it an ideal choice for those watching their calorie intake or trying to lose weight.

Rich in Antioxidants: Cucumbers and mint both contain antioxidants that help protect the body from oxidative stress and inflammation.

Detoxification: The combination of cucumber and mint can aid in detoxifying the body by flushing out toxins and promoting healthy liver function.

Digestive Health: Mint is known for its soothing effects on the digestive system. It can ease gas, bloating, and indigestion.

Skin Health: Cucumbers are high in silica and antioxidants, which contribute to healthy, glowing skin. Staying hydrated with cucumber water can also help keep your skin moisturized and clear.

Weight Management: Water consumption prior to meals can help curb hunger and avoid overindulging. The addition of cucumbers and mint makes this water more appealing, encouraging you to drink more and support weight management efforts.

Fresh Breath: Mint is a natural breath freshener. Drinking mint-infused water can help combat bad breath and promote oral hygiene.

Cucumber Mint Water is a delightful and healthful beverage that can easily be incorporated into your daily routine. Its refreshing taste and numerous health benefits make it a superior choice for staying hydrated and supporting overall well-being. Enjoy this infused water as a tasty alternative to sugary drinks and benefit from the natural goodness it provides.

Dr. Julie S. Clay

Green Tea with Lemon

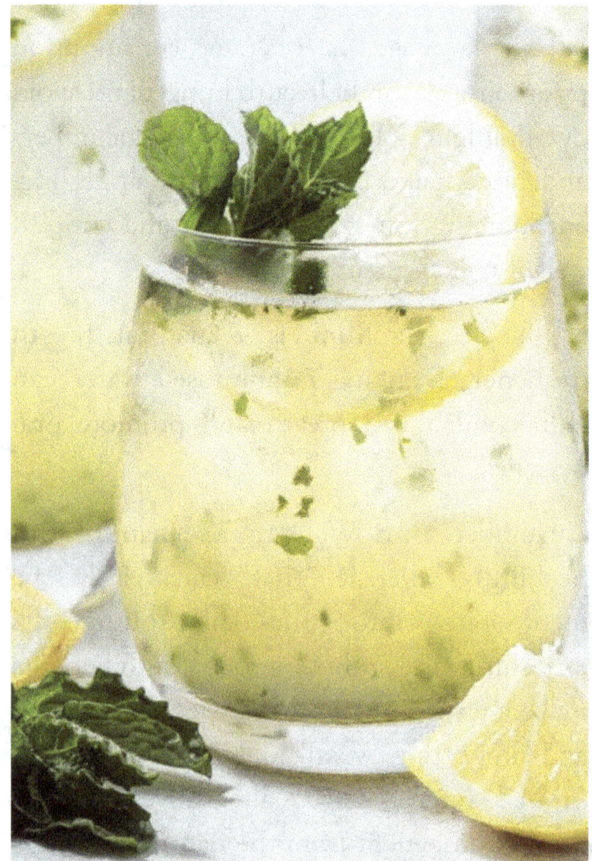

Green Tea with Lemon is a rejuvenating and flavorful beverage that combines the antioxidant-rich properties of green tea with the tangy zest of fresh lemon. This soothing drink is not only delicious but also offers a myriad of health benefits. From boosting metabolism to supporting heart health and providing a refreshing energy boost, green tea with lemon is a versatile drink that can be enjoyed hot or cold, any time of day.

Preparation Time and Serving Units

Preparation Time: 5 minutes

Cooking Time: 5 minutes (optional, for hot tea)

Servings: 2 cups

Ingredients

- 2 green tea bags or 2 teaspoons loose green tea leaves
- 2 cups (480ml) water
- 1 lemon, sliced
- Honey or sweetener of choice (optional)

Procedures

Boil Water: If making hot tea, bring 2 cups of water to a boil in a kettle or saucepan.

Steep Tea: Place the green tea bags or loose tea leaves in a teapot or heatproof pitcher. Pour the hot water over the tea and let it steep for 3-5 minutes, depending on your desired strength.

Add Lemon: While the tea is steeping, slice the lemon into thin rounds. Add a few lemon slices to the teapot or directly into each cup.

Sweeten (Optional): If desired, add honey or sweetener of choice to taste. Stir until the sweetener is dissolved.

Serve: Pour the green tea into cups, ensuring each cup has a few lemon slices. Serve hot or allow to cool for iced tea.

Enjoy: Sip and savor the refreshing taste of green tea with lemon.

Nutritional Values (per serving, 1 cup)

Calories: 0-5

Protein: 0g

Carbohydrates: 0g

Fiber: 0g

Sugars: 0g

Fat: 0g

Saturated Fat: 0g

Sodium: 0mg

Potassium: 10mg

Vitamin C: 20% DV (from lemon)

Iron: 0% DV

Cooking Tips

Water Temperature: Green tea is delicate and can become bitter if steeped in water that is too hot. Aim for water temperature around 170-180°F (77-82°C) for optimal flavor.

Steeping Time: Steeping green tea too much might make it taste harsh. Start with 3 minutes and adjust to taste.

Fresh Lemon: Use fresh lemon slices for the best flavor and aroma. Organic lemons are preferable, especially if using the peel, to avoid pesticides.

Sweetener: Green tea with lemon is naturally refreshing, but you can add a touch of sweetness with honey, agave syrup, or stevia if desired. To fit your tastes, change the quantity.

Iced Green Tea: For iced green tea, allow the tea to cool to room temperature after steeping.

Pour over ice cubes and add lemon slices for a refreshing summer drink.

Variations: Experiment with additional ingredients like fresh ginger slices, mint leaves, or a dash of cinnamon for added flavor and health benefits.

Health Benefits

Antioxidants: Green tea is rich in antioxidants called catechins, which have been shown to reduce inflammation, protect cells from damage, and lower the risk of chronic diseases such as heart disease and cancer.

Boosts Metabolism: Green tea contains compounds that can increase metabolism and promote fat oxidation, making it a popular beverage choice for weight management and fat loss.

Heart Health: There is a link between regular green tea drinking and a decreased risk of cardiovascular disease. It might assist in lowering blood pressure, cholesterol, and enhancing general heart health.

Digestive Aid: Lemon contains citric acid, which aids in digestion and helps flush toxins from the body. Green tea with lemon can soothe the stomach and promote healthy digestion.

Immune Support: Both green tea and lemon are rich in vitamin C, which strengthens the immune system and helps protect against infections and illnesses.

Hydration: It's critical to maintain hydration for general health and wellbeing.

Green tea with lemon provides a refreshing and hydrating beverage option, perfect for replacing sugary drinks and staying hydrated throughout the day.

Mental Alertness: Green tea contains caffeine, which can help improve focus, concentration, and mental alertness. Enjoying a cup of green tea with lemon in the morning can provide a gentle energy boost without the jitters associated with coffee.

Green Tea with Lemon is a delightful and healthful beverage that offers a refreshing taste and a wealth of health benefits. Whether enjoyed hot or cold, this simple drink is a wonderful addition to any diet, providing hydration, antioxidants, and a natural energy boost. Incorporate green tea with lemon into your daily routine and reap the numerous rewards it has to offer.

Berry Infused Sparkling Water

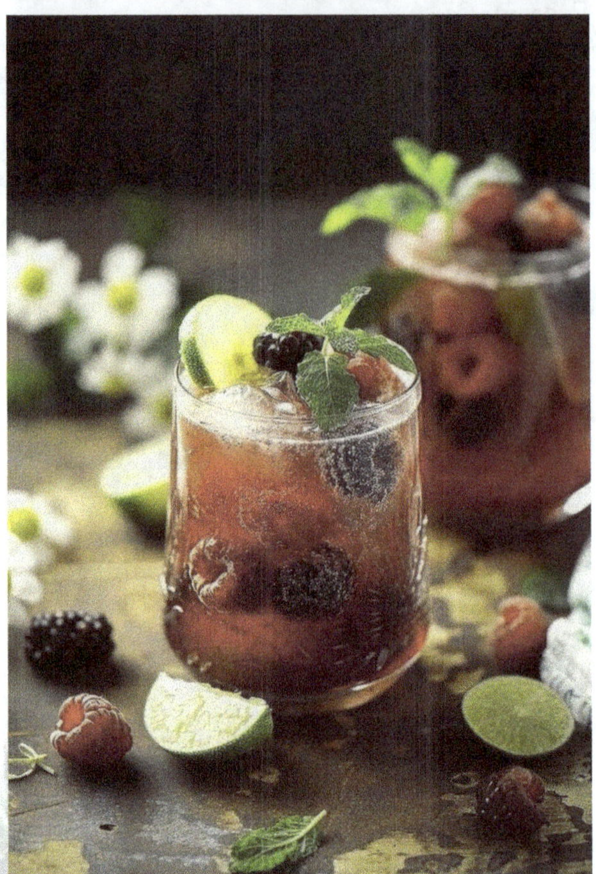

Berry Infused Sparkling Water is a refreshing and vibrant beverage that combines the natural sweetness of berries with the effervescence of sparkling water. This drink is not only delicious but also provides a burst of flavor without added sugars or artificial ingredients. It's perfect for staying hydrated and quenching your thirst on hot days or as a healthier alternative to sugary sodas and juices. With its beautiful presentation and customizable flavor combinations, berry-infused sparkling water is sure to become a favorite in your beverage repertoire.

Preparation Time and Serving Units

Preparation Time: 5 minutes

Cooking Time: None

Servings: 4 cups (1 liter)

Ingredients

- 1 cup mixed berries (such as strawberries, blueberries, raspberries, blackberries)
- 4 cups (1 liter) sparkling water
- Ice cubes (optional)
- Fresh mint leaves for garnish (optional)

Procedures

Prepare Berries: Wash the berries thoroughly under cold water and pat them dry with a paper towel. If using strawberries, hull them and slice them into halves or quarters.

Muddle Berries: In a large pitcher, gently mash the berries using a muddler or the back of a spoon. This will release their juices and enhance the flavor of the water.

Add Sparkling Water: Pour the sparkling water into the pitcher with the mashed berries. Stir gently to combine.

Serve: Fill glasses with ice cubes (if desired) and pour the berry-infused sparkling water over the ice. Garnish with fresh mint leaves for a pop of color and added freshness.

Enjoy: Sip and savor the refreshing taste of berry-infused sparkling water.

Nutritional Values (per serving, 1 cup)

Calories: 5-10

Protein: 0g

Carbohydrates: 1-2g

Fiber: 0-1g

Sugars: 1-2g

Fat: 0g

Saturated Fat: 0g

Sodium: 0mg

Potassium: 20-30mg

Vitamin C: 10-20% DV (depending on berries)

Calcium: 0% DV

Iron: 0% DV

Cooking Tips

Fresh Berries: For the greatest taste, use ripe, fresh berries. You can customize the berry combination based on your preferences and what's in season.

Muddling: Be gentle when muddling the berries to avoid breaking them down too much. The goal is to release their juices and flavor without turning them into pulp.

Sparkling Water: Choose a high-quality sparkling water with no added sugars or flavors. You can use plain sparkling water or opt for flavored varieties like lemon or lime for an extra twist.

Chill Before Serving: For optimal taste and refreshment, chill the berry-infused sparkling water in the refrigerator for at least 30 minutes before serving.

Presentation: To enhance the visual appeal of the drink, consider adding whole berries or sliced fruit to the glasses before pouring the sparkling water. This creates a beautiful presentation and adds extra flavor.

Variations: Experiment with different combinations of berries and herbs for unique flavor profiles. Try adding a few slices of cucumber or a sprig of basil or rosemary for an extra dimension of taste.

Health Benefits

Hydration: Sparkling water is hydrating, and adding berries to it can encourage you to drink more water throughout the day, helping you stay hydrated and maintain optimal bodily functions.

Antioxidants: Berries are rich in antioxidants, such as vitamin C and anthocyanins, which help protect cells from damage caused by free radicals and may reduce the risk of chronic diseases.

Low in Calories: Berry-infused sparkling water is a low-calorie beverage option, making it suitable for those watching their calorie intake or trying to manage their weight.

Vitamins and Minerals: Berries are packed with essential vitamins and minerals, including vitamin C, vitamin K, manganese, and potassium, which support immune function, bone health, and overall well-being.

Digestive Health: The fiber content in berries can aid in digestion and promote gut health. Drinking berry-infused sparkling water may help alleviate constipation and support a healthy digestive system.

Blood Sugar Control: Berries have a low glycemic index, meaning they have a minimal impact on blood sugar levels. Incorporating them into your diet, even in the form of infused water, can help stabilize blood sugar and reduce the risk of diabetes.

Natural Flavor: By infusing sparkling water with berries, you can enjoy the natural sweetness and flavor of the fruit without added sugars or artificial ingredients, making it a healthier alternative to sugary sodas and juices.

Berry Infused Sparkling Water is a delightful and healthful beverage option that offers hydration, flavor, and a dose of nutrients. Whether enjoyed on its own or as a refreshing accompaniment to meals, this drink is sure to tantalize your taste buds and leave you feeling revitalized. Experiment with different berry combinations and savor the deliciousness of this simple yet satisfying beverage.

Spiced Herbal Tea

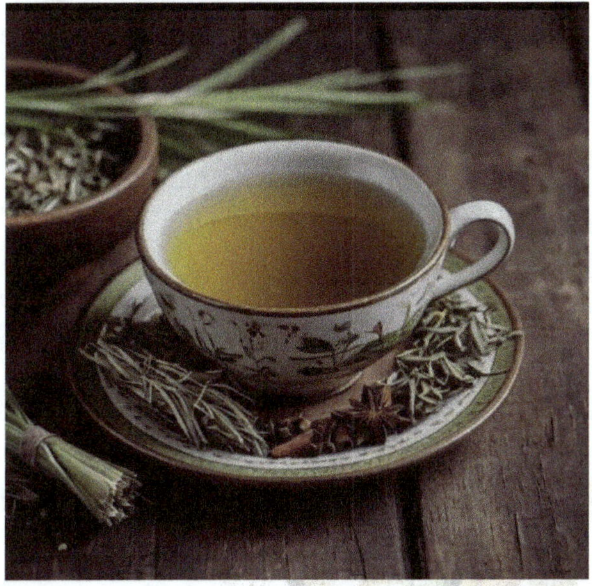

Spiced herbal tea is a comforting and aromatic beverage that combines the warmth of spices with the soothing qualities of herbal infusions. This tea is not only delicious but also offers a plethora of health benefits, making it a popular choice for relaxation, digestion, and immune support. By infusing a blend of spices and herbs in hot water, you create a fragrant and flavorful drink that can be enjoyed any time of day. Whether you're seeking a calming bedtime ritual or a soothing remedy for colds and ailments, spiced herbal tea is sure to delight your senses and nourish your body.

Preparation Time and Serving Units

Preparation Time: 5 minutes

Cooking Time: 10 minutes

Servings: 4 cups (1 liter)

Ingredients

- 4 cups (1 liter) water
- 2 cinnamon sticks
- 4 whole cloves
- 4 cardamom pods, lightly crushed
- 1-inch piece of fresh ginger, sliced
- 1 teaspoon whole black peppercorns
- 2 teaspoons loose herbal tea (such as chamomile, peppermint, or rooibos)
- Honey or sweetener of choice (optional)
- Lemon slices for garnish (optional)

Procedures

Boil Water: In a medium saucepan, bring the water to a boil over medium heat.

Add Spices: Once the water reaches a boil, add the cinnamon sticks, cloves, cardamom pods, sliced ginger, and black peppercorns to the saucepan. Reduce the heat to low and let the spices simmer for 5-7 minutes to infuse their flavors into the water.

Steep Herbal Tea: After simmering the spices, remove the saucepan from the heat. Add the loose herbal tea to the saucepan and cover with a lid. Depending on how strong you want your tea, let it steep for three to five minutes.

Strain and Serve: After steeping, strain the spiced herbal tea into cups or a teapot to remove the spices and tea leaves. Discard the solids. You can use honey or your favorite sweetener to make the tea sweeter if you'd like. Garnish with lemon slices for added flavor and visual appeal.

Enjoy: Sip and savor the comforting warmth and aromatic flavors of spiced herbal tea.

Nutritional Values (per serving, 1 cup)

Calories: 0-5

Protein: 0g

Carbohydrates: 1g

Fiber: 0g

Sugars: 0g

Fat: 0g

Saturated Fat: 0g

Sodium: 0mg

Potassium: 10mg

Vitamin C: 0% DV

Calcium: 0% DV

Iron: 0% DV

Cooking Tips

Spice Variation: Feel free to customize the spice blend according to your preferences. Other spices that work well in spiced herbal tea include star anise, fennel seeds, and cloves.

Fresh Ingredients: For the best flavor, use fresh ginger and whole spices rather than ground spices. Fresh ingredients impart a more vibrant and aromatic flavor to the tea.

Steeping Time: Adjust the steeping time based on your personal preference for tea strength. A shorter steeping time will result in a milder flavor, while a longer steeping time will yield a stronger and more intense brew.

Herbal Tea Options: Experiment with different types of herbal tea to create unique flavor profiles. Chamomile is known for its calming properties, peppermint offers a refreshing and invigorating taste, and rooibos provides a naturally sweet and nutty flavor.

Sweetening: The addition of honey or sweetener is optional and can be adjusted to suit your taste preferences. Keep in mind that some herbal teas may already have a naturally sweet flavor, so taste the tea before adding any sweeteners.

Health Benefits: While the spices in spiced herbal tea offer a myriad of health benefits, the specific benefits may vary depending on the ingredients used. Generally, spices like cinnamon, cloves, ginger, and black pepper are known for their anti-inflammatory, digestive, and immune-boosting properties.

Health Benefits

Digestive Aid: Many of the spices used in spiced herbal tea, such as ginger, cinnamon, and cardamom, have been traditionally used to aid digestion, alleviate bloating, and reduce gastrointestinal discomfort.

Anti-inflammatory: Ginger and cinnamon are potent anti-inflammatory agents that may help reduce inflammation in the body, making spiced herbal tea a soothing beverage for those with inflammatory conditions.

Immune Support: Certain spices, including ginger and cloves, possess antimicrobial properties that may help support the immune system and ward off infections, particularly during cold and flu season.

Relaxation: Chamomile tea, often used as the base for spiced herbal tea blends, is renowned for its calming and sedative effects. Enjoying a cup of spiced herbal tea before bedtime can promote relaxation and improve sleep quality.

Antioxidants: Many of the spices and herbal teas used in spiced herbal tea are rich in antioxidants, which help neutralize free radicals and protect against oxidative stress, reducing the risk of chronic diseases and promoting overall health.

Hydration: Herbal tea is an excellent way to increase fluid intake and stay hydrated throughout the day, especially for those who prefer non-caffeinated beverages or are sensitive to caffeine.

Spiced herbal tea is a versatile and healthful beverage that offers a delightful blend of flavors and numerous wellness benefits. Whether enjoyed as a warming winter drink, a soothing remedy for digestive woes, or a calming bedtime ritual, spiced herbal tea provides comfort and nourishment for both body and soul. Incorporate this aromatic brew into your daily routine and experience the joy of sipping on a cup of wellness-enhancing goodness.

30-Day Meal Plan

Week 1:
Day 1:
Breakfast: Blueberry Almond Overnight Oats
Lunch: Mediterranean Chickpea Salad
Dinner: Grilled Lemon Herb Chicken with Vegetable Stir-Fry and Brown Rice
Snack: Hummus and Veggie Platter
Day 2:
Breakfast: Avocado Toast with Poached Eggs
Lunch: Lentil and Quinoa Stuffed Peppers
Dinner: Baked Salmon with Asparagus
Snack: Kale Chips with Sea Salt
Day 3:
Breakfast: Quinoa Breakfast Bowl with Fresh Berries
Lunch: Turkey and Avocado Spinach Salad
Dinner: Quinoa and Black Bean Stuffed Zucchini
Snack: Sweet Potato Fries
Day 4:
Breakfast: Greek Yogurt Parfait with Honey and Nuts
Lunch: Beef and Broccoli Bowls
Dinner: Spinach and Feta Breakfast Wraps
Snack: Mixed Berry Fruit Salad
Day 5:
Breakfast: Tomato Basil Soup with Whole Grain Bread
Lunch: Greek Yogurt with Honey and Pistachios

Dinner: Grilled Chicken and Veggie Wraps
Snack: Roasted Garlic Brussels Sprouts
Week 2:
Day 6:
Breakfast: Strawberry Banana Smoothie
Lunch: Quinoa and Black Bean Stuffed Zucchini
Dinner: Beef and Broccoli Bowls
Snack: Hummus and Veggie Platter
Day 7:
Breakfast: Chia Seed Pudding with Fresh Mango
Lunch: Mediterranean Chickpea Salad
Dinner: Lentil and Quinoa Stuffed Peppers
Snack: Kale Chips with Sea Salt
Day 8:
Breakfast: Avocado Toast with Poached Eggs
Lunch: Turkey and Avocado Spinach Salad
Dinner: Grilled Lemon Herb Chicken with Vegetable Stir-Fry and Brown Rice
Snack: Sweet Potato Fries
Day 9:
Breakfast: Blueberry Almond Overnight Oats
Lunch: Greek Yogurt Parfait with Honey and Nuts
Dinner: Spinach and Feta Breakfast Wraps
Snack: Mixed Berry Fruit Salad
Day 10:
Breakfast: Quinoa Breakfast Bowl with Fresh Berries

Lunch: Beef and Broccoli Bowls
Dinner: Baked Salmon with Asparagus
Snack: Roasted Garlic Brussels Sprouts
Week 3-4: (Following similar pattern as Week 1 and 2)

Continue rotating between the provided recipes, ensuring a balance of nutrients and flavors each day. Feel free to mix and match meals according to your preferences while maintaining the principles of the DASH diet. Remember to stay hydrated throughout the day and listen to your body's hunger and fullness cues. Enjoy your delicious and nutritious meals!

Conclusion

Bringing It All Together

In this DASH Diet Cookbook, we've embarked on a flavorful journey toward better health and well-being. By embracing the Dietary Approaches to Stop Hypertension (DASH) principles, we've explored a variety of delicious and nutritious recipes designed to nourish both body and soul. As we conclude this culinary adventure, let's reflect on the key takeaways and how they can guide us toward a healthier lifestyle.

Recap of DASH Diet Benefits

The DASH diet is not just a temporary fix; it's a sustainable way of eating that promotes long-term health and vitality. By emphasizing whole foods rich in nutrients and minimizing processed and high-sodium foods, the DASH diet offers a multitude of benefits, including:

Lowered Blood Pressure: The DASH diet has been scientifically proven to reduce blood pressure levels, making it an effective tool for managing hypertension and improving cardiovascular health.

Improved Heart Health: With its focus on fruits, vegetables, lean proteins, and whole grains, the DASH diet supports heart health by reducing the risk of heart disease, stroke, and other cardiovascular conditions.

Weight Management: By emphasizing portion control, balanced nutrition, and mindful eating, the DASH diet can help individuals achieve and maintain a healthy weight over time.

Enhanced Nutrient Intake: The abundance of fruits, vegetables, whole grains, and lean proteins in the DASH diet ensures that you're getting a wide array of essential nutrients, vitamins, and minerals to support overall health and well-being.

Tips for Sustained Success

As you continue your journey with the DASH diet, here are some tips to help you maintain success and stay on track:

Plan Ahead: Take time to meal plan and prep your meals in advance to avoid last-minute decisions and unhealthy choices.

Stay Hydrated: To maintain proper biological processes and stay hydrated, sip on lots of water throughout the day.

Mindful Eating: Eat mindfully by focusing on your body's signals of hunger and fullness, enjoying every bite, and putting an end to outside distractions when you're eating.

Be Flexible: While the DASH diet provides guidelines for healthy eating, it's important to be flexible and adaptable to accommodate individual preferences and lifestyle factors.

Moderation is Key: Enjoy all foods in moderation, including occasional treats and indulgences, while prioritizing nutrient-dense foods the majority of the time.

Stay Active: Incorporate regular physical activity into your routine to complement your healthy eating habits and support overall well-being.

Final Thoughts and Encouragement

As you embark on your journey with the DASH diet, remember that every small step toward healthier eating habits is a step in the right direction. Whether you're just starting out or have been following the DASH diet for years, know that every meal you prepare using these recipes is a testament to your commitment to better health.

Embrace the diversity of flavors and ingredients in these recipes, and let them inspire you to get creative in the kitchen. Celebrate your progress, no matter how small, and be proud of the positive changes you're making for yourself and your loved ones.

Above all, remember that the DASH diet is not a restrictive or punitive way of eating—it's a celebration of nourishing foods and a commitment to self-care. Keep exploring, keep experimenting, and keep nourishing your body and soul with the wholesome and delicious meals found within the pages of this cookbook.

Here's to your health, happiness, and continued success on your journey with the DASH diet. Bon appétit!